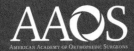

Basic Life Support (BLS) for the Health Care Provider

Meets CPR and ECC Guidelines

SIXTH EDITION

Author

Stephen J. Rahm, NRP

Medical Editors

Alfonso Mejia, MD, MPH, FAAOS

Andrew N. Pollak, MD, FAAOS

Jacqueline A. Nemer, MD, FACEP

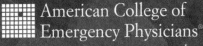
American College of
Emergency Physicians®
ADVANCING EMERGENCY CARE

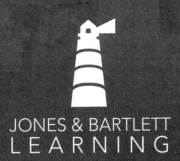
JONES & BARTLETT
LEARNING

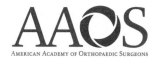

AMERICAN ACADEMY OF ORTHOPAEDIC SURGEONS

World Headquarters
Jones & Bartlett Learning
5 Wall Street
Burlington, MA 01803
978-443-5000
info@jblearning.com
www.jblearning.com

Editorial Credits
Chief Commercial Officer: Anna Salt Troise, MBA
Director, Publishing: Hans J. Koelsch, PhD
Senior Manager, Editorial: Lisa Claxton Moore
Senior Editor: Steven Kellert

AAOS Board of Directors, 2020—2021
President: Joseph A. Bosco III, MD, FAAOS
First Vice President: Daniel K. Guy, MD, FAAOS
Second Vice President: Felix H. Savoie III, MD, FAAOS
Treasurer: Alan S. Hilibrand, MD, MBA, FAAOS
Past President: Kristy L. Weber, MD, FAAOS
Chair, Board of Councilors: Thomas S. Muzzonigro, MD, FAAOS
Chair-Elect, Board of Councilors: Wayne A. Johnson, MD, FAAOS

Secretary, Board of Councilors: Claudette M. Lajam, MD, FAAOS
Chair, Board of Specialty Societies: C. Craig Satterlee, MD, FAAOS
Chair-Elect, Board of Specialty Societies: Kevin D. Plancher, MD, MPH, FAAOS
Secretary, Board of Specialty Societies: Alexandra E. Page, MD, FAAOS
Lay Member: James J. Balaschak
Members-At-Large:
    Matthew P. Abdel, MD, FAAOS
    James R. Ficke, MD, FAAOS, FACS
    Rachel Y. Goldstein, MD, MPH, FAAOS
    Alexander Vaccaro, MD, MBA, PhD, FAAOS
Chief Executive Officer (Ex-Officio): Thomas E. Arend, Jr, Esq, CAE

Substantial discounts on bulk quantities of Jones & Bartlett Learning publications are available to corporations, professional associations, and other qualified organizations. For details and specific discount information, contact the special sales department at Jones & Bartlett Learning via the above contact information or send an email to specialsales@jblearning.com.

Jones & Bartlett Learning books and products are available through most bookstores and online booksellers. To contact Jones & Bartlett Learning directly, call 800-832-0034, fax 978-443-8000, or visit our website, www.jblearning.com.

Production Credits
VP, Product Development: Christine Emerton
Director of Product Management: Jonathan Epstein
Product Manager: Carly Mahoney
Content Strategist: Ashley Procum
Project Manager: Jessica deMartin
Digital Project Specialist: Rachel DiMaggio
Director of Marketing Operations: Brian Rooney
VP, Manufacturing and Inventory Control: Therese Connell

Composition: S4Carlisle Publishing Services
Project Management: S4Carlisle Publishing Services
Cover Design: Scott Moden
Text Design: Scott Moden
Senior Media Development Editor: Troy Liston
Rights Specialist: Rebecca Damon
Cover Image (Title Page, Part Opener, Chapter Opener):
    © Jones & Bartlett Learning
Printing and Binding: LSC Communications

Library of Congress Cataloging-in-Publication Data
Names: Rahm, Stephen J., author. | Mejia, Alfonso (Orthopedic surgeon),
    editor. | Pollak, Andrew N., editor. | Nemer, Jacqueline A., editor.
Title: Basic life support (BLS) for the health care provider / author,
    Stephen J Rahm ; medical editors, Alfonso Mejia, Andrew N. Pollak,
    Jacqueline A. Nemer.
Other titles: Health care provider CPR.
Description: Sixth edition. | Burlington, MA : Jones & Bartlett Learning,
    [2022] | Preceded by Health care provider CPR / [edited by] Benjamin
    Gulli, Jacqueline A. Nemer, Jeanne A. Noble, Stephen J. Rahm. Fifth
    edition. [2017]. | Includes bibliographical references and index. |
    Summary: " This manual is developed for use within health care provider
    level (both pre-hospital and in-hospital) CPR training courses offered
    through the Emergency Care & Safety Institute. This title is ideal for
    use within courses designed to certify health care providers in CPR and
    AED. The content of this manual has been updated to meet or exceeds the
    2020 scientific recommendations developed by the International Liaison
    Committee on Resuscitation (ILCOR) and is consistent with the CPR and
    ECC Guidelines as established by the American Heart Association (AHA)
    and other resuscitation councils around the world"-- Provided by
    publisher.
Identifiers: LCCN 2020055191 | ISBN 9781284228946 (paperback)
Subjects: MESH: Cardiopulmonary Resuscitation--methods | Handbook
Classification: LCC RC87.9 | NLM WG 39 | DDC 616.1/025--dc23
LC record available at https://lccn.loc.gov/2020055191

6048

Printed in the United States of America
25 24 23 22   10 9 8 7 6 5 4 3 2

Brief Contents

Contents

Welcome to the Emergency Care & Safety Institute

Welcome to the Emergency Care & Safety Institute (ECSI), brought to you by the American Academy of Orthopaedic Surgeons (AAOS) and the American College of Emergency Physicians (ACEP).

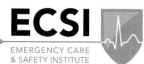

ECSI is an internationally renowned organization that provides training and certifications that meet job-related requirements as defined by regulatory authorities such as the Occupational Safety and Health Administration (OSHA), The Joint Commission, and state offices of EMS, Education, Transportation, and Health. Our courses are delivered throughout a range of industries and markets worldwide, including colleges and universities, business and industry, government, public safety agencies, hospitals, private training companies, and secondary school systems.

ECSI programs are offered in association with the AAOS and ACEP. AAOS, the world's largest medical association of musculoskeletal specialists, is known as the original name in EMS publishing with the first EMS textbook ever in 1971, and ACEP is widely recognized as the leading name in all of emergency medicine.

ECSI Course Catalog

Individuals seeking training from ECSI can choose from among various traditional classroom-based courses or alternative online courses such as:

- Advanced Cardiac Life Support (ACLS)
- Babysitter Safety
- Basic Life Support (BLS) and Cardiopulmonary Resuscitation (layperson and health care provider levels)
- Bloodborne and Airborne Pathogens
- Driver Safety
- Emergency Medical Responder
- First Aid (standard, advanced, pediatric, wilderness, sports, pet)
- And more!

ECSI offers a wide range of textbooks, instructor and student support materials, and interactive technology, including online courses. ECSI student manuals are the center of an integrated teaching and learning system that offers resources to better support instructors and train students. The instructor supplements provide practical hands-on, time-saving tools such as PowerPoint presentations, skills demonstration videos, and web-based distance learning resources. Technology resources provide interactive exercises and simulations to help students become prepared for any emergency.

Documents attesting to ECSI's recognitions of satisfactory course completion will be issued to those who successfully meet the course requirements. Written acknowledgement of a participant's successful course completion is provided in the form of a Course Completion Card, issued by the Emergency Care & Safety Institute.

Visit **www.ECSInstitute.org** today!

2020 Guideline Updates and the COVID-19 Pandemic

This book meets and exceeds the 2020 American Heart Association (AHA) Emergency Cardiovascular Care (ECC) Guidelines and the 2020 International Liaison Committee on Resuscitation (ILCOR) Consensus on Science with Treatment Recommendations (CoSTR). At the time of this edition's development, we find ourselves in the middle of a 100-year event: the COVID-19 pandemic. These updates were made with the COVID-19 pandemic in mind.

Although we are perhaps more mindful than ever of the importance of personal protective equipment (PPE) in our profession, readers will still notice some variability throughout this textbook with regard to PPE worn by health care providers as they care for patients. They may also question the inclusion of skills and techniques that are discouraged in the context of COVID-19.

We have tried throughout the text to apply the best current knowledge and practices available. However, that science is developing rapidly. We will make every attempt to make supplemental material available that reflects the most updated knowledge.

Personal Protective Equipment

Prior to 2020, the level of PPE commonly worn by all health care providers during treatment typically included gloves. Eye protection was added during situations when the risk of a splash was high or when there was significant risk of aerosolization of material that could potentially come in contact with the eyes. For example, eye protection was typically worn while caring for patients who were bleeding significantly, when performing airway-related procedures, and during maternity calls. It was added on calls when there was a perceived high risk of being splashed with a potentially contaminated bodily fluid. In the COVID-19 era and beyond, however, use of eye protection has become more common.

In addition, face masks are now standard equipment for all interpersonal encounters, not just patient encounters. At various times throughout the pandemic, masks have been required in public places, such as grocery stores. In many locations, masks are mandatory when social distancing is not possible. Simple face masks or cloth masks decrease the risk of infection for the person wearing the mask and decrease the risk associated with viral shedding that is a known consequence of infection, even in asymptomatic hosts. In other words, people without symptoms can still be infected with the virus and thus transmit it to others. Asking everyone to wear a mask in public can make the environment safer.

Furthermore, it is recommended that providers caring for COVID-19 patients or those who have overt symptoms, such as fever or cough, wear a higher level of protection, such as an N95 respirator. There is variability in that recommendation also, as many agencies are using N95 respirators for all patient encounters, given the increased level of protection afforded and the pervasiveness in the population of asymptomatic individuals who could transmit the disease.

Cardiopulmonary Resuscitation

While incorporating best practices in an evolving pandemic, we must remain true to the education standards for the health care provider and the often less-than-ideal conditions in which they work. This book has followed the widely accepted guidelines of the American Heart Association. The use of mouth-to-mouth rescue breathing and mouth-to-barrier and mouth-to-mask devices are included in these standards. The use of a bag-mask device, while included in this book and strongly encouraged in the context of active community transmission of an aerosolized disease, may not be available to all health care providers. Further more, many health care providers carry limited or no first aid supplies. To present bag-mask ventilation as the only method of rescue breathing is to deprive them of any method of providing rescue breathing. These techniques are still key competencies for the health care provider.

Art and Photos

Revising the illustrations and images throughout the book has been a challenge. Organizing photo shoots has been dramatically hindered by necessary social distancing restrictions. For this reason, we ensured that first aid providers and other relevant parties are wearing face masks and appropriate eye protection in any new images that were shot for this textbook. However, we were not able to update all photos to reflect new practice guidelines. It is certainly our hope that by the time the next edition is published, our knowledge of best practices with regard to PPE will be more static and there will be more consistency in the appearance of PPE in images throughout the text.

Acknowledgments

The authors, the medical editors, the Jones & Bartlett Learning Public Safety Group, the American Academy of Orthopaedic Surgeons, and the American College of Emergency Physicians would like to thank all of the reviewers that generously offered their time, expertise, and talent to the making of this sixth edition.

Reviewers

J. Adam Alford, NRP
VCU Center for Trauma and Critical Care
    Education
Richmond, Virginia

Mark A. Boisclair, MPA, NRP
EMS Program Instructor
Chattahoochee Valley Community College
Phenix City, Alabama

Kent Courtney
Paramedic, Fire Fighter, Rescue Technician,
    Educator
Essential Safety Training and Consulting
Lake Montezuma, Arizona

Chance Cummings
Lieutenant, Paramedic, EMS Liaison Officer
Starkville Fire Department
Starkville, Mississippi

James W. Fogal, NRP, MA
Auburn University
Auburn, Alabama

Fidel O. Garcia
Paramedic
Professional EMS Education
Grand Junction, Colorado

**Michele M. Hoffman, MS, Ed,
RN, NREMT**
James City County Fire Department
Williamsburg, Virginia

Joe Kalilikani Jr., BAS, EMT
Pasadena City College
Pasadena, California

Gregory S. Neiman, MS, NRP, NCEE
EMS Liaison
Virginia Commonwealth University Health
Richmond, Virginia

William H. Turner, MS, NRP, EMSI
Assistant Professor, Program Director of
    Emergency Medical Technology
Shawnee State University
Portsmouth, Ohio

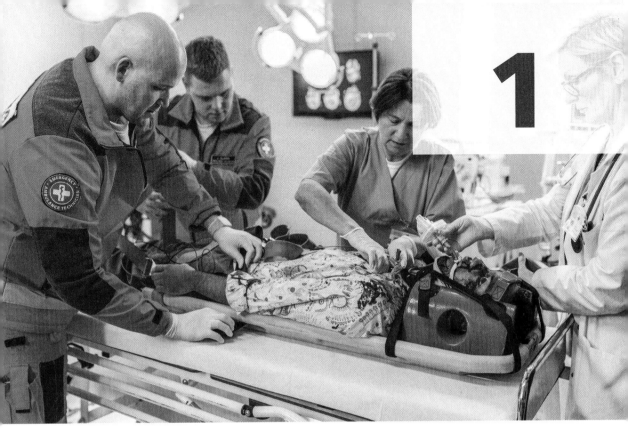

Emergency Cardiac Care and the Health Care Provider

Health Care Providers as Rescuers

Health care providers will likely participate in many cardiac arrest resuscitations during their careers—not only while on duty but potentially during off-duty activities around the community. A patient's cardiac arrest may be attributed to ventricular fibrillation (VF), acute myocardial infarction (AMI), poisoning or overdose, stroke, or trauma, among other causes.

Most cardiac arrests are not witnessed by health care providers working in the hospital or prehospital setting; they typically occur before a health care provider arrives at the scene or reaches the patient's side. When at work, health care providers should follow current, evidence-based national guidelines, as well as their local protocols, for providing basic and advanced cardiac life support.

Health care providers share a defined duty to respond to an emergency. They are found in a broad range of health care, allied health care, and nonmedical settings **FIGURE 1-1**. Examples of professionals who function as health care providers include:

- Firefighters
- Law enforcement officers
- Emergency medical services (EMS) personnel—emergency medical responders (EMRs), emergency medical technicians (EMTs), advanced emergency medical technicians (AEMTs), and paramedics
- Nurses, nurse practitioners, physicians, and physician assistants
- Dentists and dental assistants
- Occupational or physical therapists and laboratory technicians
- Industrial and business personnel
- Park services personnel
- Ski patrol personnel
- Lifeguards
- Airline personnel
- Cruise ship personnel

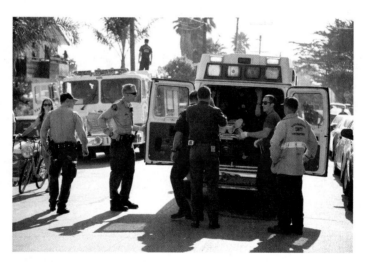

FIGURE 1-1 Health care providers include professionals from many fields: EMS personnel, firefighters, law enforcement officials, and physicians.
© VDB Photos/Shutterstock.

The initial care that these personnel provide plays an important role in the outcome of a patient and is known as **basic life support (BLS)**. Three of the most important BLS skills are rescue breathing, cardiopulmonary resuscitation (CPR), and the Heimlich maneuver:

- Rescue breathing is provided when someone has stopped breathing **FIGURE 1-2**.

- CPR is provided when someone's heart has stopped beating **FIGURE 1-3**.
- The Heimlich maneuver is performed when someone has an airway obstruction (choking) **FIGURE 1-4**.

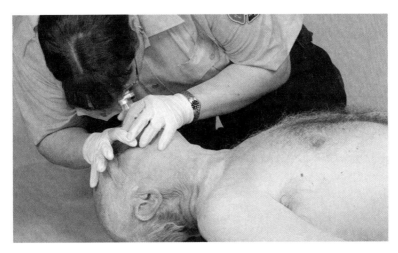

FIGURE 1-2 Seal your mouth over the mouthpiece and begin rescue breathing.
© Jones & Bartlett Learning. Courtesy of MIEMSS.

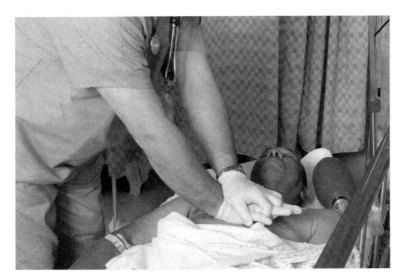

FIGURE 1-3 Perform chest compressions.
© Jones & Bartlett Learning. Courtesy of MIEMSS.

This manual covers these and other skills used to care for people experiencing respiratory and cardiac emergencies. It also covers special situations you may encounter and the use of specialized equipment, most notably automated external defibrillators (AEDs) **FIGURE 1-5**.

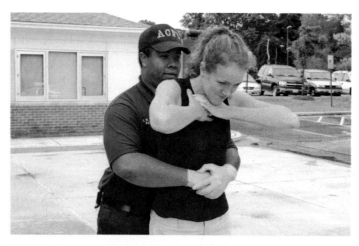

FIGURE 1-4 Apply abdominal thrusts (Heimlich maneuver).
© Jones & Bartlett Learning. Courtesy of MIEMSS.

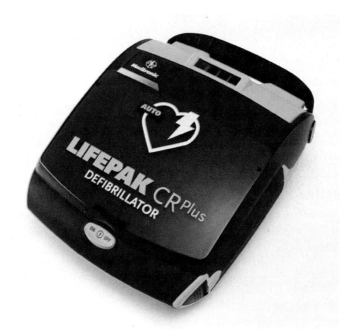

FIGURE 1-5 Automated external defibrillators have a built-in rhythm analysis system to determine whether the patient needs to be shocked.
Courtesy of Physio-Control, Inc.

Preparing for Emergencies

As a health care provider, you need to prepare for an emergency in advance. Reading this text and taking a CPR course are only the first steps in preparing for the various emergency situations you could encounter. You will need additional physical and mental preparation before you will be ready to provide emergency care. This preparation includes:

- Being physically fit for the strenuous work you will perform
- Being mentally prepared for the challenges you could face
- Periodically reviewing your skills and rehearsing your response with other health care providers
- Practicing with the equipment and supplies you will be using
- Examining additional reference material, as it becomes available, to stay up to date on changes in CPR techniques and advances in emergency care
- Being prepared for the personal risks associated with your job, such as the possibility of injury or disease transmission

---

FYI

Emergency Cardiac Care

In some instances, the level of emergency cardiac care (ECC) that you provide may require additional education or certification. Subjects covered in this education may include advances in the treatment of cardiac and respiratory arrest, the use of specific equipment designed for either hospital or nonhospital settings, and advanced life support techniques used by other members of the emergency care team. Members of the ECC team include EMTs, paramedics, nurses, nurse practitioners, physician assistants, and physicians.

In addition, you can help implement an effective ECC system in your community. You can educate the public about how to prevent heart disease; teach people to recognize the signs of cardiac arrest; emphasize the importance of calling for assistance (9-1-1); encourage others to learn BLS skills, such as CPR; and advocate for public access defibrillation (PAD).

SOFT SKILL

Team-Based Resuscitation

For health care providers who routinely care for patients with life-threatening respiratory or cardiovascular emergencies, it is imperative to have a plan of action *before* the emergency occurs. This can include giving your team members preassigned tasks (eg, airway management, chest compressions, defibrillation). If each team member knows their assignment ahead of time, then the "time to intervention" is reduced. Practice running "codes" with preassigned roles to maximize your team's readiness and have a more efficient resuscitation.

Disease Transmission and Precautions

As a health care provider, you must be aware of the risks of disease transmission associated with emergency care. The infectious diseases you will encounter range in severity from mild to life threatening. The following bloodborne and airborne diseases are of particular concern to health care providers:

- Hepatitis B and hepatitis C (bloodborne)
- Human immunodeficiency virus (HIV) (bloodborne)
- Tuberculosis (airborne)
- Severe acute respiratory syndrome coronavirus 2019 (SARS-CoV-19) (airborne)

Hepatitis

Hepatitis is a viral infection of the liver. The virus can stay in the liver and cause severe damage (cirrhosis) and cancer. Hepatitis B and hepatitis C are most worrisome to health care providers. A different virus causes each type of hepatitis. According to the Centers for Disease Control and Prevention (CDC), an estimated 862,000 people in the United States have chronic hepatitis B infection.

A vaccine for hepatitis B is available and recommended for all health care providers. Federal laws require employers to offer the vaccine to employees who may be at risk of exposure. People who have not received the vaccine and who are exposed to hepatitis B may begin to experience signs and symptoms within 2 weeks to 6 months. The signs and symptoms of hepatitis B resemble those of the flu and include fatigue, nausea, loss of appetite, abdominal pain, and jaundice (yellowing of the skin). Although some people with hepatitis B may not have the usual signs and symptoms, they can still infect others who are exposed to their blood. Like hepatitis B, hepatitis C can lead to long-term liver disease, including cancer. Although there is currently no vaccine for hepatitis C, advances have been made in its treatment.

FYI

Hepatitis B Vaccine

According to the CDC, the hepatitis B vaccine provides greater than 90% protection to infants, children, and adults who receive the three-shot immunization series before being exposed to the virus.

Human Immunodeficiency Virus

Human immunodeficiency virus (HIV) attacks white blood cells and destroys the body's ability to fight infection. Acquired immunodeficiency syndrome (AIDS) is the most advanced stage of HIV infection. Like hepatitis, HIV is transmitted through blood contact; it is also spread through contact with other body secretions (ie, semen, vaginal secretions). According to the CDC, an estimated 1.2 million people in the United States were infected with HIV at the end of 2018, the most recent year for which this information is available. Approximately 14% (or 1 in 7) of these individuals are unaware of their infection. With proper treatment, many people can live for decades with HIV infection; however, when HIV infection progresses to AIDS, the disease is nearly always fatal. Because there is no HIV vaccine, the best defense is to avoid direct contact with blood.

Tuberculosis

Airborne diseases are viruses and bacteria introduced into the air by coughing or sneezing. Tuberculosis (TB) is a serious disease that affects the respiratory system. It is caused by bacteria that settle in the lungs. The signs and symptoms of TB include coughing, fatigue, weight loss, chest pain, and coughing up blood. A strain of TB known as multidrug-resistant TB has been identified. It is resistant to the two strongest medications used to treat TB. Currently there is no TB vaccine available in the United States.

Severe Acute Respiratory Syndrome Coronavirus 2 (SARS-CoV-2)

A new virus appeared in late 2019, and in a short period of time became a global pandemic. The virus, called severe acute respiratory syndrome coronavirus 2 (SARS-CoV-2), causes an infection called coronavirus disease 2019 (COVID-19). SARS-CoV-2 is spread by aerosolized respiratory particles, and although it primarily affects the lungs, it can also affect other body systems. In most people infected with the virus, signs and symptoms develop within 2 to 14 days. This can include fever, cough, headache, body aches, fatigue, and a loss of taste and/or smell. Some people infected with SARS-CoV-2 are asymptomatic carriers and may never become ill, although they may still be able to transmit the virus to others. Illness severity can range from mild symptoms to respiratory system failure and death. People older than 65 years, especially those with underlying medical problems such as hypertension, heart disease, and diabetes, are at greatest risk for severe illness and death.

Although face coverings, such as surgical masks, do not stop SARS-CoV-2 particles, they do help reduce the chance of an infected person spreading the virus to other people by reducing the number of respiratory droplets emitted during coughing or talking.

Protection

Taking standard precautions means creating a barrier between you and the patient by using personal protective equipment (PPE). The standard equipment you should have before responding to a cardiac or respiratory emergency includes:

- Eye protection, such as goggles or eyeglasses with side shields
- Medical exam gloves, such as latex, vinyl, or nitrile gloves
- Mouth-to-barrier devices for rescue breathing **FIGURE 1-6**
- Antiseptic wipes or solution for washing your hands immediately after providing care

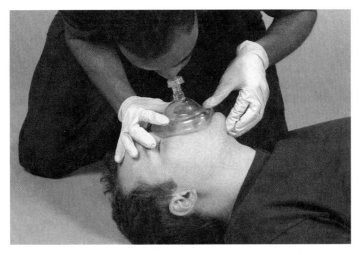

FIGURE 1-6 A barrier device is an essential component of your PPE.
© Jones & Bartlett Learning. Courtesy of MIEMSS.

As a health care provider, you are eligible to receive vaccinations against certain types of disease as outlined by federal and state Occupational Safety and Health Administration (OSHA) regulations. Your employer is also required to establish work practices and engineering controls to help reduce the likelihood of disease transmission. OSHA's regulations apply to those people who are designated or expected to render care as part of their job. They exclude unassigned employees who provide unanticipated care.

Cardiovascular Disease: Improving the Odds

Cardiovascular disease (CVD) is a spectrum of disease processes affecting the heart and circulatory system. According to the 2020 Heart and Stroke Statistical Update by the American Heart Association, the death rate from CVD in the United States is 219.4 per 100,000 people. On average, someone dies from CVD every 37 seconds, with an estimated 2,353 deaths per day or approximately 860,000 deaths per year. Almost half of these deaths are due to fatal heart attacks attributed to coronary artery disease (CAD). Many fatal heart attacks could be prevented each year through a heart-healthy lifestyle that reduces the risk of heart disease. Each year, CAD causes approximately 360,000 cases of sudden cardiac arrest (SCA) in an out-of-hospital setting, usually within the first few hours of the onset of signs and symptoms. SCA is a condition in which the heart suddenly and unexpectedly stops beating. When this happens, blood stops flowing to the brain and other vital body organs; death usually occurs if SCA is not treated within minutes.

Although the death rate from CVD has declined slightly, there is still much room for improvement. Many of the causes leading to SCA could be prevented through a heart-healthy lifestyle that reduces the risks of heart disease. As a health care provider, you have an obligation to reduce your personal risk factors as well as to educate others so that they might reduce their risk factors.

Risk Factors

Risk factors for CVD fall into two categories: modifiable and nonmodifiable. Modifiable risk factors are behaviors or conditions that can be controlled, such as cigarette smoking, high blood pressure, high cholesterol, lack of exercise, stress, and obesity. Nonmodifiable risk factors are those that cannot be controlled, such as sex, age, and heredity. Cigarette smokers are much more likely to experience the development of CVD, suffer a heart attack, or have a stroke compared to nonsmokers. The risk increases with the number of cigarettes smoked, and the risk decreases, and may even be eliminated over time, if the person stops smoking.

High blood pressure, left untreated, significantly increases the chances of CAD and is a major risk factor for a stroke. Fortunately, there are numerous medications available to control high blood pressure.

High cholesterol can result from a diet high in saturated fats. A fatty diet has been associated with the development of fatty deposits on the artery walls (atherosclerosis). Countries, such as the United States, where the average person's diet is high in saturated fats have correspondingly high rates of CAD.

Lack of exercise and a sedentary lifestyle make the body ill prepared for physically demanding tasks that can raise a person's heart rate above tolerable levels and increase stress on the heart. Obesity is also a high-risk factor, not only because it is often associated with poor diet and lack of exercise but also because excessive weight strains the heart.

Prevention: Heart-Healthy Living

A commitment to a heart-healthy lifestyle is the best way to prevent CVD and heart attack. The basics of heart-healthy living are easy to remember and simple to teach to others in your community. As a health care provider, you are responsible for educating others about prevention practices and for being a role model to others by practicing prevention.

- Stop smoking and urge others to stop.
- Exercise regularly. A brisk 20- to 30-minute walk every day provides excellent aerobic conditioning.
- Eat a healthy, balanced diet, low in sodium and saturated fat.

- Have your blood pressure checked regularly and take prescribed medication for high blood pressure.
- Maintain a healthy body mass index (BMI).

SOFT SKILL

Maintaining Clinical Competence

When a person takes a CPR course, they are said to be "trained." However, such training simply gives the provider the core knowledge on best resuscitation practices at the time they attended the training. In order to maintain clinical competence, it is important to keep up to date with the latest recommendations regarding best practices in resuscitation science and procedures. This may be accomplished by reading peer-reviewed journal publications, research papers, or other reliable sources of information.

The Chain of Survival

The number of deaths from SCA can be reduced if a timely and specific sequence of events, called the chain of survival, takes place. Although the general principles of care for cardiac arrest are the same, the pathway of care for a person experiencing out-of-hospital cardiac arrest (OHCA) differs from that of a person experiencing in-hospital cardiac arrest (IHCA). Therefore, separate chains of survival—each consisting of six links—have been identified for the two settings. The OHCA chain of survival describes the importance of early activation of the emergency response system, care initiated by the bystander, care provided by EMS personnel (ie, EMTs and paramedics) until the patient arrives at the hospital, and recovery of the cardiac arrest survivor **FIGURE 1-7**. The IHCA chain of survival describes the sequence of care that begins with early recognition and prevention of cardiac arrest; an integrated system of care provided by physicians, nurses, and respiratory therapists if cardiac arrest occurs; and recovery of the cardiac arrest survivor **FIGURE 1-8**.

Prevention, Early Recognition, and Activation of the Emergency Response System

In the hospital setting, a system of surveillance (ie, rapid response or early warning system) should be in place to prevent cardiac arrest. If cardiac arrest occurs in the hospital, the code team must be activated. Code teams are composed of physicians, nurses, respiratory therapists, and technicians. They are often linked by a unified paging system; each member carries a digital pager and/or is notified by an overhead paging system. Team members can be at the patient's side within minutes.

In the prehospital setting, access the EMS system by calling 9-1-1. According to the National Emergency Number Association, the 9-1-1 system covers approximately 96% of the U.S. population. Those without 9-1-1 service must access EMS by calling their local emergency response number. A prompt call will ensure the timely arrival of EMS personnel with the necessary training and equipment to provide appropriate care.

The dispatcher who takes emergency calls should be trained to recognize SCA, as well as the signs and symptoms of other respiratory and cardiac emergencies. This knowledge will enable them to provide

OHCA

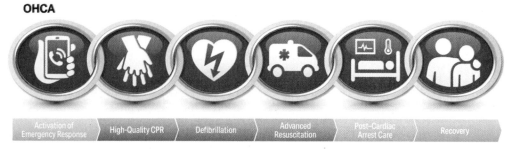

FIGURE 1-7 Chain of survival for out-of-hospital cardiac arrest (OHCA).
Reprinted with permission Circulation.2020;142:S366-S468 ©2020 American Heart Association, Inc

prearrival instructions to callers over the phone while the EMS personnel is en route. In addition to instructing a caller on how to perform CPR and remove an airway obstruction, dispatchers should advise callers with symptoms of a cardiac emergency, who have no history of aspirin allergy or active or recent gastrointestinal bleeding, to chew and swallow 160 to 325 mg of aspirin. Early administration of aspirin has proven to be effective in reducing mortality from heart attacks.

Immediate High-Quality CPR

When a person's heart stops beating, cardiopulmonary resuscitation (CPR) is needed. CPR temporarily helps circulate oxygenated blood throughout the body. This sustained oxygen circulation lessens the chance of brain injury and increases the chance of survival—especially when CPR is coupled with early defibrillation. To be most effective, CPR must be started promptly and performed correctly. Each minute of delay reduces the chance of survival. Limiting interruptions in CPR is absolutely critical; if CPR must be interrupted, the interruption should last no longer than 10 seconds. Advanced cardiac life support (ACLS) interventions (ie, cardiac rhythm checks, advanced airway management, medication administration) should be planned to allow maximum chest compression time.

Rapid Defibrillation

Ventricular fibrillation (VF), a chaotic "quivering" of the heart caused by an abnormality in the heart's electrical conduction system, is the most common initial heart rhythm found in SCA. Conversion of VF to a normal heart rhythm requires electrical defibrillation; CPR alone cannot correct it. Even with the most effective CPR, a person's chance of survival is poor unless they also receive early defibrillation. When defibrillation is delivered within the first minute following SCA, the incidence of return of spontaneous circulation can be very high. However, as SCA persists, the chance that defibrillation will be successful diminishes rapidly.

Although manual defibrillators are available for rapid deployment in the hospital setting and in EMS systems that provide advanced life support, they are not available to the public. Therefore, public access defibrillation (PAD) using AEDs is strongly supported. Several states have enacted legislation regarding the use of AEDs by trained rescuers and bystanders. When applied to a patient in cardiac arrest, AEDs can reliably identify abnormal cardiac rhythms, such as VF, and advise the operator to deliver a shock to correct the rhythm. Because AEDs are both simple to operate and economical, their use could save many lives through early defibrillation.

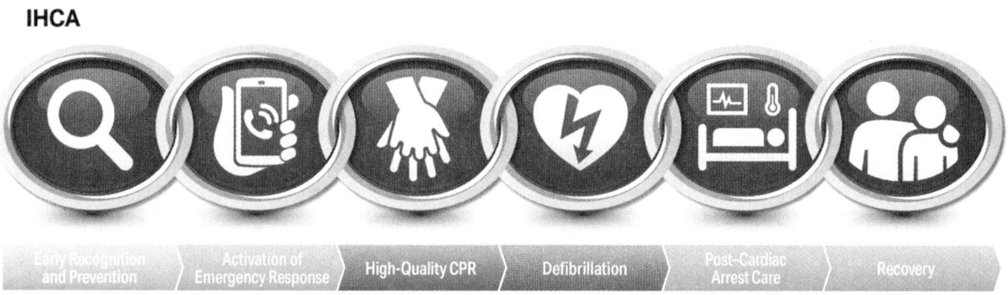

IHCA

FIGURE 1-8 Chain of survival for in-hospital cardiac arrest (IHCA).
Reprinted with permission Circulation.2020;142:S366-S468 ©2020 American Heart Association, Inc

Basic and Advanced Resuscitation

Basic and advanced resuscitation describes care provided by EMTs and paramedics before the patient arrives at the hospital. In addition to continuing high-quality CPR, the following care can be provided by EMS personnel:

- BLS
- Basic and advanced airway management
- ACLS, which includes manual defibrillation, vascular access, and medication administration
- Transport of the patient to an appropriate hospital, such as a designated resuscitation center, for further treatment

Postcardiac Arrest Care

After the patient is stabilized in the emergency department, further cardiopulmonary and neurologic support is provided to improve the patient's recovery. This support can include:

- Additional medication therapy to support blood pressure
- Targeted temperature management
- Maintenance of blood glucose levels
- Cardiac catheterization
- Detection and treatment of seizures
- Admission to the intensive care unit for additional critical care management

Recovery

The ultimate goal of resuscitation is to return a patient to their preevent state as a functional individual. Patients who are successfully resuscitated from cardiac arrest and survive can face many challenges following the event. In addition to physical challenges, survivors can experience cognitive and emotional challenges that can take months to years to resolve. This link in the chain of survival emphasizes that these patients may require ongoing therapies or interventions to assist them in their recovery. This may include physical or occupational therapy or psychological support.

Early Warning Signs of a Heart Attack

Heart attacks are the number one cause of death in the United States. Some people die because they ignore or downplay the early warning signals. Most of the damage to the heart occurs in the first 2 hours. For this reason, people experiencing a heart attack need rapid medical care to help minimize the amount of damage to the heart. But because the early warning signals are often mild, they are not easily recognized by laypeople as potentially fatal, and people delay seeking the necessary care. It is also important to note that females—particularly older females—may not experience classic symptoms of a heart attack; this is especially true when they have a history of diabetes. Their symptoms may consist only of unexplained nausea, generalized weakness, or a general sense of not feeling well.

Part of your responsibility as a health care provider is to educate community members about the importance of recognizing a heart attack in its early stages so that immediate action can be taken to save more lives.

Early warning signals of a heart attack include:
- Chest discomfort characterized by any of the following:
  - Recurs and increases in intensity
  - Becomes more intense with exertion and diminishes with rest
  - Is accompanied by lightheadedness, fainting, sweating, nausea, or shortness of breath
  - Is present hours or even days before the chest pain becomes severe
- A burning sensation in the chest or throat (often confused with heartburn or indigestion)
- Pain that radiates down the arm, across the shoulders, jaw, and neck or into the back

The public should be educated to:
- Recognize the early signals of a heart attack in another person and intervene.
- Convince any family member, friend, coworker—even a stranger—who exhibits signs of a heart attack that medical care is needed immediately.
- Move from being passive observers and listeners to active, early heart attack care providers.

As professionals, you can educate people in your community and encourage them to act:
- The progression of a heart attack can be halted if people are alert to the early signals and actively intervene.
- It makes sense to have mild chest discomfort evaluated before a complete coronary artery blockage occurs and damages the heart.
- Once the heart stops, it may be restarted through defibrillation. But by that time, heart damage has already occurred and sometimes death cannot be prevented.
- Denial and delay are common among people experiencing signs of a heart attack and are often reinforced by those around the person. Reasons for this unfortunate response include:
  - The reality of a heart attack is too traumatic to face.
  - A heart attack poses serious short- and long-term inconveniences to the person and the person's family.

- A heart attack is inconsistent with the person's self-perception or the bystander's perceptions of the person.
- People often believe that a heart attack is something that happens to others, not to themselves or their loved ones.
- Use the mnemonic ACT WISELY to teach others how to intervene:
  A: Acknowledge that there is an issue.
  C: Calmly assess the situation and persuade the person to get help.
  T: Tenacity. Be persistent, and do not give in.
  W: Willingness. Be willing to act.
  I: Influence and use your skills creatively.
  S: Simplify the discussion and decisions.
  E: Empathy. Understand why the person is resisting help.
  L: Link the person with the nearest hospital.
  Y: "Yes, I will get help!" Get the person to state this.

Legal and Ethical Considerations

Modern CPR techniques were developed and advocated 60 years ago. CPR instruction has become an accepted part of the health care system, in both medical and nonmedical settings. As litigation has increased so has awareness of ethical and legal concerns involving CPR. Health care providers need to understand these issues as well as their rights and responsibilities **FIGURE 1-9**.

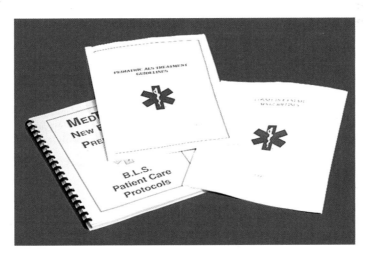

FIGURE 1-9 Protocol books.
© Jones & Bartlett Learning. Courtesy of MIEMSS.

Duty to Act

Generally speaking, the duty of any health care provider is to have the knowledge ordinarily possessed and to exercise the skill and care ordinarily used by trained and skilled members of the same profession in the same or similar circumstances. The duty of a health care provider, therefore, is to practice their profession as any other health care provider would.

Duty to act is a concept that defines the circumstances in which a health care provider is legally obligated to provide assistance to a person in need. It considers questions such as is a health care provider obligated to help 24 hours a day, whether on duty or not? And, does a health care provider–patient relationship ever extend beyond the scope of employment? These questions are not easily answered and often depend on factors such as the terms of a provider's employment, the context of the emergency at hand, and local and/or state regulations.

Standard of Care

The quality of the care you provide to people is based on training standards, laws, and the specifications of authorities, such as national organizations, that guide practice in your profession. This expected quality is commonly referred to as the standard of care. If you fail to perform according to this expected norm, you may be subject to legal action.

Consent

A competent person—that is, a person who is of legal age and has decision-making capacity—has the right to refuse or limit medical treatment, even if this refusal could shorten their life. A patient's right to choose among various treatment options—including no treatment—depends on their capacity to give consent, or permission to treat. Informed consent exists when the patient agrees to treatment and understands the significance of the situation as well as the risks and benefits of accepting medical care.

Because informed consent is not possible if a person is unconscious, incapacitated, or otherwise unable to make a rational decision, the concept of implied consent is used. In these situations, it is assumed (implied) that the patient would consent to lifesaving care if they could do so.

Protected Health Information

As a health care provider, you are legally obligated to safeguard a patient's protected health information (PHI) under the Health Insurance Portability and Accountability Act (HIPAA). This means that you cannot release a patient's PHI, such as their name, Social Security number, medical history, and other personally identifiable information, without their expressed consent. The only individuals to whom you can release such information are other health care providers who will be directly involved in the continuation of care.

Advance Directives

Efforts have been directed at allowing people to make decisions before a crisis occurs. An informed decision that is made in advance of an emergency is popularly termed an advance directive. Living wills, Physician Orders for Life-Sustaining Treatment (POLST) forms, and durable powers of attorney for health care are examples of advance directives.

Although advance directives may be useful to you, their reliability and availability at the time of need may vary dramatically. You should familiarize yourself with the standards of practice and legal requirements in your area. Although conversations between a patient and their family, friends, or physicians can help guide decisions, legal decisions by patients and health care providers require written directives. Local practice statutes or regulations may define the acceptability of various forms of advance directives.

Written advance directives are, from a legal standpoint, the most desirable form of consent. To avoid confusion, a number of states and local health care systems have developed standard formats for advance directives in their regions. This standardized approach allows rescuers to identify and implement valid directives quickly.

Withholding or Discontinuing CPR

CPR is not always appropriate. The traditional contraindications to starting CPR are incineration, decapitation, and clear signs of prolonged death, such as rigor mortis, the stiffening of the body, or dependent lividity, when the blood settles to the lowest point of the body. The indications to stop CPR are rescuer exhaustion; a direction to stop from a physician; or relief of duty by another, equally trained person(s). Recently, these guidelines have been reconsidered based on an increased role by the patient receiving care in medical decision-making and a reassessment of the futility of CPR in certain circumstances.

Currently, CPR can be withheld or discontinued if it is not consistent with the patient's wishes, is not in the patient's best interest, or is not medically indicated. Some specific situations in which CPR may not be indicated include cardiac arrest due to trauma (injury) with an extended response time, situations in which the provider's personal safety is threatened, and situations in which written protocols, called do-not-resuscitate (DNR) orders, result in a decision that CPR should not be initiated **FIGURE 1-10**.

Emotional Support for the Family

Despite your best efforts, resuscitation attempts are not always successful. The notification of family members of the death of their loved one is an important component of the resuscitation. Notification should be given as compassionately as possible so that the family members understand that BLS and ACLS efforts failed and that the patient has died. Avoid using expressions such as "passed on"; be direct and concise. Consider the family's religious beliefs, and, if appropriate, enlist the help of clergy members. Also consider cultural practices of the family.

Additionally, some reports suggest that it may be beneficial for family members to be present during a resuscitation attempt; however, many family members will not request to be present unless asked by the health care provider. The health care provider and the resuscitation team must be sensitive to the presence of family members in the room.

Good Samaritan Laws

Good Samaritan laws exist in all states. They provide legal immunity and minimize liability in situations where rescuers act in good faith, within the scope of their training and without compensation, and where no negligence exists. Because the precise wording of these laws varies from state to state, you must understand what protection the laws of your state afford you.

Figure: 25 TAC §157.25 (h)(2)

OUT-OF-HOSPITAL DO-NOT-RESUSCITATE (OOH-DNR) ORDER
TEXAS DEPARTMENT OF STATE HEALTH SERVICES

This document becomes effective immediately on the date of execution for health care professionals acting in out-of-hospital settings. It remains in effect until the person is pronounced dead by authorized medical or legal authority or the document is revoked. Comfort care will be given as needed.

STOP DO NOT RESUSCITATE

Person's full legal name _____   Date of birth _____   ☐ Male ☐ Female

A.   Declaration of the _adult person_: I am competent and at least 18 years of age. **I direct that none of the following resuscitation measures be initiated or continued for me: cardiopulmonary resuscitation (CPR), transcutaneous cardiac pacing, defibrillation, advanced airway management, artificial ventilation.**

Person's signature _____   Date _____   Printed name _____

B.   Declaration by _legal guardian, agent or proxy_ on behalf of the adult person who is incompetent or otherwise incapable of communication:

I am the: ☐ legal guardian;   ☐ agent in a Medical Power of Attorney; OR   ☐ proxy in a directive to physicians of the above-noted person who is incompetent or otherwise mentally or physically incapable of communication.

Based upon the known desires of the person, or a determination of the best interest of the person, **I direct that none of the following resuscitation measures be initiated or continued for the person: cardiopulmonary resuscitation (CPR), transcutaneous cardiac pacing, defibrillation, advanced airway management, artificial ventilation.**

Signature _____   Date _____   Printed name _____

C. Declaration by a _qualified relative_ of the adult person who is incompetent or otherwise incapable of communication: I am the above-noted person's:

☐ spouse,   ☐ adult child,   ☐ parent, OR   ☐ nearest living relative, and I am qualified to make this treatment decision under Health and Safety Code §166.088.

To my knowledge the adult person is incompetent or otherwise mentally or physically incapable of communication and is without a legal guardian, agent or proxy. Based upon the known desires of the person or a determination of the best interests of the person, **I direct that none of the following resuscitation measures be initiated or continued for the person: cardiopulmonary resuscitation (CPR), transcutaneous cardiac pacing, defibrillation, advanced airway management, artificial ventilation.**

Signature _____   Date _____   Printed name _____

D. Declaration by _physician based on directive to physicians by a person now incompetent or nonwritten communication to the physician by a competent person_: I am the above-noted person's attending physician and have:

☐ seen evidence of his/her previously issued directive to physicians by the adult, now incompetent; OR   ☐ observed his/her issuance before two witnesses of an OOH-DNR in a nonwritten manner.

I direct that none of the following resuscitation measures be initiated or continued for the person: cardiopulmonary resuscitation (CPR), transcutaneous cardiac pacing, defibrillation, advanced airway management, artificial ventilation.

Attending physician's signature _____   Date _____   Printed name _____   Lic# _____

E. Declaration on behalf of the _minor person_: I am the minor's: ☐ parent;   ☐ legal guardian; OR   ☐ managing conservator.

A physician has diagnosed the minor as suffering from a terminal or irreversible condition. **I direct that none of the following resuscitation measures be initiated or continued for the person: cardiopulmonary resuscitation (CPR), transcutaneous cardiac pacing, defibrillation, advanced airway management, artificial ventilation.**

Signature _____   Date _____

Printed name _____

TWO WITNESSES: (See qualifications on backside.) We have witnessed the above-noted competent adult person or authorized declarant making his/her signature above and, if applicable, the above-noted adult person making an OOH-DNR by nonwritten communication to the attending physician.

Witness 1 signature _____   Date _____   Printed name _____

Witness 2 signature _____   Date _____   Printed name _____

Notary in the State of Texas and County of_____. The above noted person personally appeared before me and signed the above noted declaration on this date:_____.

FIGURE 1-10 Do-not-resuscitate (DNR) form.
Courtesy of Texas Department of State Health Services.

PREP KIT

Ready for Review

- As a health care provider, you are likely to be involved in the treatment of people with cardiac emergencies. Your ability to provide these people with appropriate and effective BLS is an essential skill.
- Although prevention remains critical to reducing cardiac incidents, emergency cardiac care is essential in sustaining life once an incident does occur.
- Emergency cardiac care includes providing CPR and other emergency care procedures to people experiencing cardiac and respiratory arrest. The chain of survival includes steps that are essential to effective emergency cardiac care for people experiencing out-of-hospital cardiac arrest and in-hospital cardiac arrest.
- Except in very specific situations, health care providers are required to perform CPR and other BLS procedures. Advance directives are a form of informed consent, made prior to an emergency situation, that enable a person to indicate, verbally or in writing, that they do not want to receive CPR. Unless you have a reliable advance directive or are able to determine through specific criteria that CPR would be futile for the person or dangerous to yourself or others, you should initiate CPR.

Vital Vocabulary

acquired immunodeficiency syndrome (AIDS) A disease in which the body's immune system loses its ability to fight infections and disease processes. It is caused by infection with the human immunodeficiency virus.

advance directive Written documentation that a competent patient uses to specify medical treatment should that person become unable to make decisions in the future; also called a living will.

advanced cardiac life support (ACLS) The administration of intravenous fluids and medications to help resuscitate a patient experiencing cardiac arrest and prevent a recurrence of cardiac arrest.

atherosclerosis A disease characterized by a thickening and destruction of the arterial walls, caused by fatty deposits within them; the arteries lose their ability to dilate and carry oxygen-enriched blood.

automated external defibrillator (AED) A device that detects treatable, life-threatening cardiac arrhythmias (ventricular fibrillation and ventricular tachycardia) and delivers the appropriate electrical shock to the patient.

basic life support (BLS) Noninvasive emergency lifesaving care that is used to treat medical conditions, including airway obstruction, respiratory arrest, and cardiac arrest.

cardiopulmonary resuscitation (CPR) A method of temporarily circulating oxygenated blood throughout the body of a patient experiencing cardiac arrest. It combines rescue breathing and chest compressions.

cardiovascular disease (CVD) A spectrum of disease processes affecting the heart and circulatory system; the leading cause of death in the United States.

PREP KIT continued

chain of survival A sequence of events that, if performed in a timely manner, can improve survival from cardiac arrest; it includes early recognition and prevention, activation of the emergency response system, immediate high-quality CPR, rapid defibrillation, basic and advanced resuscitation, postcardiac arrest care at the hospital, and recovery of the cardiac arrest survivor.

consent Permission to treat given by the patient to the health care provider.

coronary artery disease (CAD) The presence of atherosclerosis in the coronary arteries, which may cause symptoms such as angina or acute myocardial infarction (heart attack).

coronavirus disease 2019 (COVID-19) The respiratory disease caused by the SARS-CoV-2 virus.

defibrillation Use of a special electrical current in an attempt to convert a fibrillating (chaotically beating) heart to a normal, rhythmic beat.

dependent lividity Blood settling to the lowest point of the body, causing discoloration of the skin.

duty to act The job-defined, legal obligation to provide care.

Good Samaritan laws Laws that protect a person from legal liability when providing emergency care, in good faith, to a suddenly ill or injured person.

hepatitis A viral infection of the liver.

human immunodeficiency virus (HIV) A virus that attacks white blood cells and destroys the body's ability to fight infection. Acquired immunodeficiency syndrome results from HIV infection.

implied consent The assumption that a patient would give consent for treatment if they were able to do so.

informed consent Consent to treatment given by the patient who understands the risks and benefits of accepting treatment.

manual defibrillators Devices that display the patient's cardiac rhythm on a screen and enable the provider to manually select the energy setting before delivering a shock.

personal protective equipment (PPE) Equipment that protects its wearer, according to standard precautions, from potentially contagious bloodborne or airborne diseases.

public access defibrillation (PAD) An initiative that provides training to the public about the importance of early defibrillation and makes automated external defibrillators available in the community for rapid deployment by bystanders.

rigor mortis Stiffening of the body; a definitive sign of death.

severe acute respiratory syndrome coronavirus 2 (SARS-CoV-2) The virus that causes an infection called coronavirus disease 2019 (COVID-19), which primarily affects the lungs and can lead to respiratory failure and death.

standard of care The quality of care provided to people based on training standards, laws, and national organizations.

standard precautions An infection control concept and practice that assumes all body fluids are potentially infectious; infectious exposures are dealt with by creating a barrier between the rescuer and the person receiving care.

sudden cardiac arrest (SCA) A condition in which the heart suddenly and unexpectedly stops beating. When this happens, blood stops flowing to the brain and other vital organs; death usually occurs if SCA is not treated within minutes.

PREP KIT continued

tuberculosis (TB) A disease affecting the respiratory system that is caused by bacteria that settle in the lungs.

ventricular fibrillation (VF) Disorganized, ineffective twitching of the ventricles, resulting in no blood flow and a state of cardiac arrest.

Check Your Knowledge

1. Signs and symptoms of hepatitis include:

   A. difficulty breathing and chest pain.

   B. loss of appetite, fatigue, and jaundice.

   C. vomiting of blood, pale skin, and nausea.

   D. headache, severe weakness, and dehydration.

2. Which of the following is a modifiable risk factor for cardiovascular disease?

   A. Sex

   B. Heredity

   C. Age

   D. High cholesterol

3. The chance of survival for a patient in cardiac arrest is maximized if:

   A. CPR and defibrillation are provided within a few minutes after the onset of cardiac arrest.

   B. an ACLS provider arrives at the patient's side and administers medications within 10 minutes.

   C. their body is cooled while chest compressions and rescue breaths are in progress.

   D. any health care provider arrives and begins care within 5 minutes after the onset of cardiac arrest.

4. Which of the following statements regarding ventricular fibrillation (VF) is correct?

   A. Manual defibrillators are preferred over automated external defibrillators when treating VF.

   B. VF is the most common rhythm found in sudden cardiac arrest and is treated with defibrillation.

   C. Most people who present with VF are older than 70 years and have numerous medical conditions.

   D. CPR alone will often correct VF and should be performed for 5 minutes before defibrillation is attempted.

5. Which of the following statements regarding a patient's consent to treatment is correct?

   A. Consent to treat is implied if the patient is competent and of legal age.

   B. A competent adult patient has the right to refuse treatment, even if the refusal may shorten their lifespan.

   C. A patient's right to choose among various treatment options depends on their ability to give implied consent.

   D. If a patient is unconscious, the health care provider should assume that the patient would not wish to be treated.

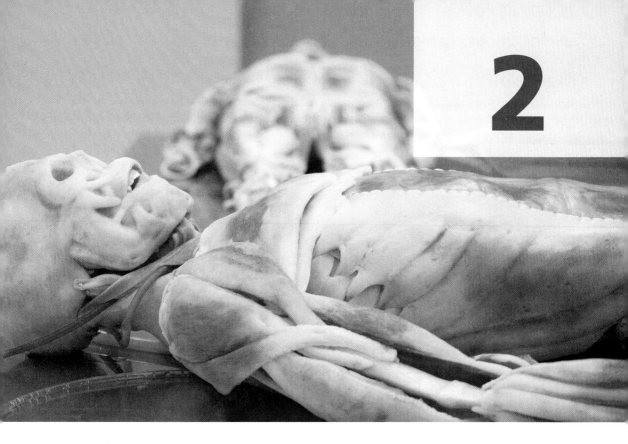

2

Understanding the Human Body

Body Systems

Failure of any body system causes serious medical conditions. The inability of one or more of these systems to function properly can lead to death. The challenge for the health care provider is to provide basic life support (BLS) to keep their patient alive and correct conditions resulting from the failure of these body systems. This chapter discusses a basic overview of the body systems so that you can better understand their interrelationships when providing care. For example, if the respiratory system fails, the nervous and cardiovascular systems will be deprived of oxygen. If the nervous system, specifically the brain, is without oxygen, the patient will lose consciousness. If the heart is without oxygen, it will fail to function. Similarly, failure of the cardiovascular system to circulate oxygen throughout the body will cause the other body systems to collapse.

The Respiratory System

Oxygen is the body's most vital external resource required to sustain life. The respiratory system delivers oxygen to the lungs and removes waste products such as carbon dioxide **FIGURE 2-1**. Because the body is unable to store oxygen for more than a few minutes, the respiratory system must function continuously. If it stops for any reason, such as during drowning or choking, the body will die within minutes.

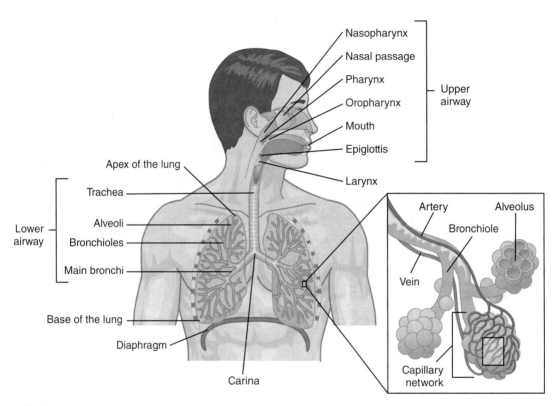

FIGURE 2-1 Human respiratory system.
© Jones & Bartlett Learning.

Structure and Function

During breathing, air enters the mouth and nose, where it is warmed, cleaned, and humidified. It passes through the pharynx (throat) and past the epiglottis, a flap of cartilage that covers the glottis (the opening to the trachea) during swallowing, thus preventing food and liquids from entering the lungs. Air enters the trachea (windpipe), which branches into two main passages called bronchi that enter each lung. Each bronchial tube divides into increasingly smaller tubes (bronchioles), ending in alveoli (air sacs) enclosed in tiny blood vessels called capillaries. This is where oxygen and carbon dioxide are exchanged—a process called pulmonary respiration **FIGURE 2-2**.

Air enters and is expelled from the lungs through the actions of the intercostal muscles (muscles of the chest wall) and the diaphragm, a dome-shaped, sheetlike muscle that separates the chest cavity from the abdomen. During inhalation (drawing air into the lungs), the diaphragm contracts, moving

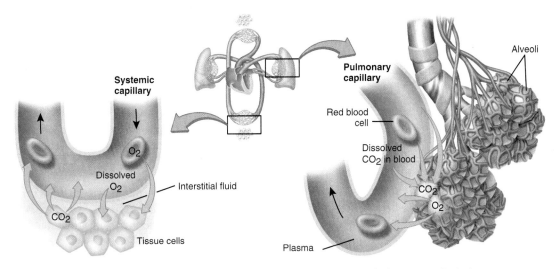

FIGURE 2-2 The exchange of carbon dioxide (CO_2) and oxygen (O_2) in the lungs (pulmonary respiration).
© Jones & Bartlett Learning.

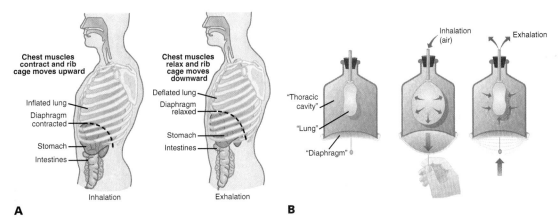

FIGURE 2-3 A. Chest muscle and diaphragm contractions. **B.** The function of the diaphragm can be illustrated by a balloon in a bell jar, with a rubber diaphragm at the bottom. If the diaphragm is pulled downward, air will flow into the balloon.
© Jones & Bartlett Learning.

downward and flattening, and the intercostal muscles contract, moving the ribs upward and outward. As the chest expands, the pressure inside the chest cavity becomes less than the pressure outside the body. This creates a vacuum, which pulls air in and expands the lungs to equalize the pressure. When the diaphragm and intercostal muscles relax, they force the air out (**exhalation**) in the same amount as was initially inhaled **FIGURE 2-3**. Adults normally breathe 12 to 20 breaths per minute (respiratory rate). Normal breathing rates for children are 12 to 40 breaths per minute (depending on age), and infant breathing rates are 30 to 60 breaths per minute.

Normal breathing is an automatic process that occurs in response to the body's need for oxygen. Specialized areas of the brain sense the levels of oxygen and carbon dioxide in the blood and regulate the breathing rate and depth (deep, normal, or shallow) to maintain an appropriate balance of these gases.

The Cardiovascular System

The cardiovascular system is composed of the heart and blood vessels. It functions to deliver oxygen and nutrients throughout the body and to remove carbon dioxide and other metabolic waste.

Structure and Function

A person's heart is about the size of their fist. The heart lies behind and slightly to the left of the lower sternum (breast bone), between the lungs, and in front of the esophagus (food tube to the stomach) and the trachea. The heart muscle (myocardium) is essentially a double pump with four chambers: the right and left atria and the right and left ventricles. The left and right sides of the heart are separated by a wall called the septum. The right side of the heart receives oxygen-poor venous blood from the body through two large veins called the venae cavae. This blood enters the right atrium and is pumped to the right ventricle and then to the lungs, where carbon dioxide in the blood is exchanged for oxygen. The oxygen-rich blood returns to the left atrium of the heart, which pumps it to the left ventricle and then throughout the body FIGURE 2-4.

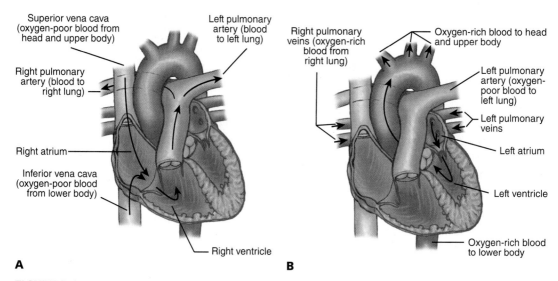

FIGURE 2-4 A. The right side, or lower-pressure side, of the heart pumps blood from the body through the lungs. B. The left side, or higher-pressure side, of the heart pumps oxygen-rich blood to the rest of the body.
© Jones & Bartlett Learning.

The heart (cardiac) muscle is unique among body tissues because it can generate its own electrical impulses without stimulation from nerves. In addition, the heart has special conduction tissue, which can rapidly transmit electrical impulses to the muscular tissue of the heart. The tissues that generate the electrical impulses are called pacemaker cells because they set the pace, or rate, for contraction of the chambers. These pacemaker cells are located in nodes throughout the heart.

The electrical impulses generated by the pacemakers can be detected and measured by an electrocardiogram (ECG). If the heart muscle is damaged by lack of blood flow and oxygen, the muscle tissue may send out abnormal electrical signals that interfere with the normal pacemaker signals. These abnormal signals can cause dysrhythmias, which can interfere with normal heart function. The most severe dysrhythmia is ventricular fibrillation (VF), a disorganized contraction of the heart in which blood is not pumped from the heart. If not corrected within a few minutes, VF leads to death. A defibrillator is used to correct this life-threatening dysrhythmia.

Blood vessels consist of arteries and arterioles, which carry oxygenated blood from the heart to the rest of the body, and veins and venules, which carry oxygen-poor blood back to the heart **FIGURE 2-5**. The pulmonary artery is a little different from other arteries because it carries oxygen-poor blood. It is still an artery because it carries blood away from the heart. The pulmonary vein carries oxygenated blood from the lungs back to the heart. Capillaries are tiny blood vessels where the exchange of oxygen for carbon dioxide and other waste occurs.

Each time the heart beats, a pressure wave of blood circulating through the arteries generates a pulse. The heart of the average adult at rest beats 60 to 100 times per minute, and the pulse can be felt at different areas of the body. The pulse felt on the thumb side of the inner wrist, alongside the radius (radial bone), is known as the radial pulse. The pulse felt on the side of the neck, over the carotid artery, is known as the carotid pulse. The pulse felt on the inside of the upper thigh, at the femoral artery, is known as the femoral pulse. Check the pulse of an unconscious (unresponsive) adult or child at the carotid artery or femoral artery. If the patient is an infant (younger than 1 year), check the pulse at the inside of the upper arm at the brachial artery (brachial pulse).

The Nervous System

The nervous system is the command center of the human body. It is controlled by the brain, which regulates both the heart rate and the respiratory rate. The nervous system allows the body to react to internal and external stimulation and controls movement. Signals travel from the brain through a network of nerves that extends down the spinal cord and branches out through the body. These nerves act much like transistor circuits, sending and receiving messages at an incredible rate of speed **FIGURE 2-6**.

Structure and Function

The brain and spinal cord serve as the headquarters and communications system for the body. They are well protected, because without them, all other systems would fail. The brain is encased in the skull, and the spinal cord is inside the vertebrae of the spine.

The spinal cord can be thought of as the main circuit board of a communications system. It relays sensory information from peripheral nerves to the brain and forwards signals from the brain to the body through motor fibers. Injury to any area of the spinal cord can disrupt the flow of information to and from the brain.

The brain has three main parts: the cerebrum (large portion of the brain), the cerebellum (small portion of the brain), and the brainstem **FIGURE 2-7**. The cerebrum controls thought, sensation, memory, and voluntary motions such as walking or picking up an object. The cerebellum is located at the back of the head and below the cerebrum. It controls balance by coordinating signals from the eyes and inner ears. The medulla oblongata, located in the brainstem, connects the cerebrum and the cerebellum to the spinal cord. It controls involuntary motions, such as breathing, heart rate, and digestion.

Of all the organs and tissues in the body, the brain is particularly sensitive to oxygen deprivation. When either the respiratory or the cardiovascular system fails, cells in the brain begin to die in as little as 4 to 6 minutes because of the lack of oxygen. Rescue breathing and cardiopulmonary resuscitation (CPR) can help keep the brain oxygenated until the patient can receive specialized medical care.

It is important to determine, whenever possible, the patient's normal level of consciousness (awareness). For example, some patients may be awake but unable to answer basic questions regarding orientation to person, place, or time. Knowing a patient's normal level of consciousness helps determine whether their current level of consciousness is a reliable indicator of injury or illness. When the brain is deprived of oxygen, the patient's level of consciousness can become altered.

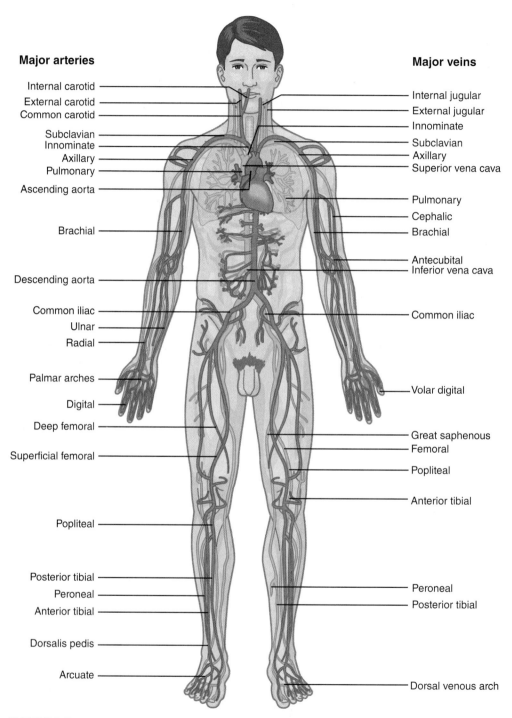

Major arteries

Internal carotid
External carotid
Common carotid
Subclavian
Innominate
Axillary
Pulmonary
Ascending aorta
Brachial
Descending aorta
Common iliac
Ulnar
Radial
Palmar arches
Digital
Deep femoral
Superficial femoral
Popliteal
Posterior tibial
Peroneal
Anterior tibial
Dorsalis pedis
Arcuate

Major veins

Internal jugular
External jugular
Innominate
Subclavian
Axillary
Superior vena cava
Pulmonary
Cephalic
Brachial
Antecubital
Inferior vena cava
Common iliac
Volar digital
Great saphenous
Femoral
Popliteal
Anterior tibial
Peroneal
Posterior tibial
Dorsal venous arch

FIGURE 2-5 Human cardiovascular system.
© Jones & Bartlett Learning.

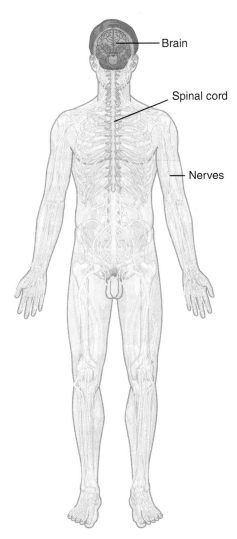

FIGURE 2-6 The human nervous system.
© Jones & Bartlett Learning.

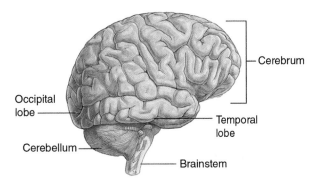

FIGURE 2-7 Surface of the brain.
© Jones & Bartlett Learning.

When Body Systems Fail

The body, particularly the brain, lungs, and heart, requires a constant supply of oxygen. Without oxygen, cells in the brain begin to die in as little as 4 to 6 minutes. Without this critical command center, the rest of the body cannot survive. The goals of CPR are to supply oxygen to the blood and to keep blood flowing to the brain until more advanced medical care is available.

Respiratory System Failure

Disease, injury, choking, drowning, or cardiac arrest can compromise respiration. For example, respiratory diseases, such as asthma, cause the airway tissues to swell, narrowing or obstructing the airway. An airway obstruction can cut off the supply of air to the lungs.

The signs and symptoms of respiratory distress include the following:

- Signs of hypoxia (low oxygen levels in the blood), which may include restlessness, anxiety, and confusion
- Signs of airway obstruction or swelling, which may include grunting, stridor (high-pitched sound during inhalation), and an inability to speak
- Flared nostrils
- Unusually rapid, deep, or irregular breathing
- Straining to breathe (use of facial and neck muscles, retraction of muscles between the ribs, tracheal tugging [collapsing of the trachea, causing it to draw back into the neck])
- Cyanosis (blue color in lighter skinned individuals and gray or whitish color in darker skinned individuals) of fingernails and around lips

The most severe sign of respiratory system failure is respiratory arrest. In this condition, breathing stops and the skin becomes cyanotic or ashen. Without rapid intervention, brain cells will die from oxygen deprivation.

Cardiovascular System Failure

Heart disease can narrow the primary blood vessels of the heart, the coronary arteries. This narrowing is referred to as coronary artery disease (CAD). When the inside of one of these arteries becomes so narrow that blood flow is restricted, oxygen delivery to the heart is diminished. This decreased oxygen in the heart can impair heart function. A mild form of diminished blood flow can result in angina.

Angina is a condition in which the heart is temporarily deprived of oxygen (ischemia) due to partial narrowing of a coronary artery. Angina usually does no permanent damage to the heart; however, it is a sign of CAD, and people with angina should seek medical attention. Stable angina occurs after a predictable amount of physical exertion; it usually lasts less than 15 minutes and is relieved by rest and/or nitroglycerin tablets or spray, which dilate (open) the coronary arteries. Unstable angina does not follow a predictable pattern; it typically occurs during periods of nonexertion (eg, sleep) and is often not relieved by rest and/or nitroglycerin.

Acute coronary syndrome (ACS) is a spectrum of clinical disease that refers to unstable angina and acute myocardial infarction (heart attack). The most common symptom of ACS is chest pain, pressure, or discomfort.

Acute Myocardial Infarction

Acute myocardial infarction (AMI), known more commonly as a heart attack, occurs when a portion of the heart muscle (myocardium) is deprived of oxygen, resulting in cell death (tissue necrosis) **FIGURE 2-8**.

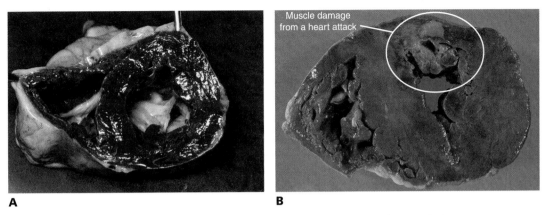

FIGURE 2-8 A. Healthy heart. **B.** Heart showing muscle damage from a heart attack due to a clot in a coronary artery.
A: © Klaus Guldbrandsen/Science Source; **B:** © Dr. E. Walker/Science Source.

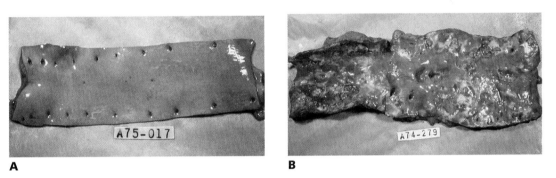

FIGURE 2-9 Inside the artery wall. **A.** Normal artery (aorta). **B.** Atherosclerotic artery.
© American Academy of Orthopaedic Surgeons.

AMI usually occurs as a result of atherosclerosis, a condition in which fatty deposits (**plaque**) significantly and acutely obstruct one or more of the coronary arteries **FIGURE 2-9**.

The following are signs and symptoms of AMI:

- Chest pain or discomfort, radiating to the arms, jaw, or upper back
- Difficulty breathing (dyspnea)
- Sweating (diaphoresis)
- Nausea or vomiting
- Irregular pulse in the presence of other signs and symptoms
- Weakness
- Cool, pale, moist skin

Not all of these signs and symptoms are present in all patients. Approximately 20% of people experiencing AMI have no chest pain, a condition sometimes called a "silent" heart attack. Other people—especially older adults, women, and people with diabetes—may experience vague or unusual symptoms such as weakness, unexplained nausea, or "not feeling well."

The signs and symptoms of AMI are similar to those of angina but are usually more intense. Chest pain associated with AMI lasts longer than 15 minutes and is usually unrelieved by rest and/or nitroglycerin. People with AMI are at risk for experiencing sudden cardiac arrest, especially within the first few hours after the onset of symptoms.

If treated in a timely fashion, permanent damage to the heart can be minimized. The patient may be taken to the cardiac catheterization lab, where the affected coronary artery can be unblocked by a procedure called angioplasty. A stent may then be placed, which keeps the coronary artery open. If the hospital does not have a catheterization lab, the patient may be eligible to receive a **fibrinolytic drug** (clot bluster)—that can dissolve the clot in the coronary artery.

Stroke

Two types of **stroke** exist: ischemic and hemorrhagic. A stroke occurs when a blood vessel in the brain delivering oxygen-rich blood becomes occluded (ischemic stroke) or a blood vessel ruptures (hemorrhagic stroke), causing the brain to receive less blood flow than it requires **FIGURE 2-10**. Approximately 87% of strokes are ischemic. Deprived of oxygen, nerve cells beyond the occluded or ruptured blood vessel cannot function and die within minutes. Because dead brain cells cannot be replaced, the devastating effects of a stroke are often permanent. According to the American Heart Association, stroke is the fifth leading cause of death in the United States.

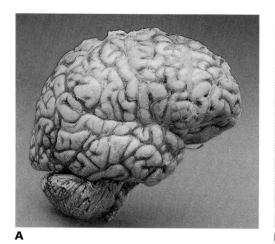
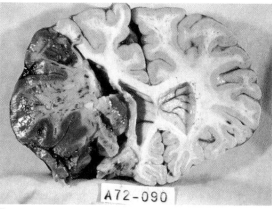

A   **B**

FIGURE 2-10 A. Healthy brain. **B.** Damage resulting from a severe stroke.
© American Academy of Orthopaedic Surgeons.

The signs and symptoms of a stroke include the following:

- Weakness, numbness, or paralysis of the face, arm, or leg on one side of the body
- Blurred or decreased vision, especially in one eye
- Difficulty speaking or understanding speech
- Dizziness or loss of balance
- Sudden, severe, and unexplained headache
- Pupils that are unequal in size

Health care providers should use stroke assessment tools, such as the Cincinnati Stroke Scale **TABLE 2-1** or the National Institutes of Health (NIH) stroke scale. These tools check for physical findings

TABLE 2-1 Cincinnati Stroke Scale

Test	Normal	Abnormal
Facial Droop (Ask patient to show teeth or smile.)	Both sides of the face move equally well.	One side of the face does not move as well as the other.
Arm Drift (Ask patient to close eyes and hold both arms out with palms up.)	Both arms move the same, or both arms do not move.	One arm does not move, or one arm drifts down compared with the other side.
Speech (Ask patient to say, "The sky is blue in Cincinnati.")	The patient uses the correct words with no slurring.	The patient slurs words, uses inappropriate words, or is unable to speak.

© Jones & Bartlett Learning.

(eg, facial droop, arm weakness/drift, speech abnormalities). Health care providers should also evaluate people for other causes of altered mental status, including seizures and hypoglycemia.

If the onset of the stroke symptoms is within the past 3 hours (4.5 hours in certain circumstances), the patient may be eligible to receive a fibrinolytic medication that can dissolve the clot in the affected cerebral artery. The longer that therapy is delayed, the greater the chance of a negative outcome. Therefore, it is imperative to recognize the signs of a stroke promptly and transport the patient as soon as possible to a designated stroke center.

Not every health care facility is capable of providing comprehensive stroke care; therefore, plans should be developed in advance for providing initial management of patients with acute stroke, as well as for timely transfer to a comprehensive stroke care facility.

PREP KIT

Ready for Review

- The body systems that are most concerning in an emergency situation are the nervous system, respiratory system, and cardiovascular system.
- The nervous system functions as the control and communications center for the body. The respiratory system supplies the body with oxygen and removes carbon dioxide. The cardiovascular system transports oxygenated blood from the lungs to the rest of the body.
- Each beat of the heart produces a pulse, which can be felt at various sites, such as the inside of the wrist (radial), the neck (carotid), and the inside of the upper arm (brachial).
- The nervous, respiratory, and cardiovascular systems depend on one another for normal function. Respiratory system failure deprives the brain and heart of oxygen. Brain cells deprived of oxygen begin to die within 4 to 6 minutes. Lack of blood flow to the heart muscle can result in permanent damage and cardiac arrest within a few minutes.
- Oxygen deprivation in the heart can lead to chest pain (angina) or AMI, commonly known as a heart attack. Oxygen deprivation of the brain can result in loss of consciousness. A stroke occurs when blood vessels delivering oxygen-rich blood to the brain rupture or become blocked so that part of the brain does not get the necessary blood flow. Nerve cells that are deprived of oxygen cannot function and die within minutes. The devastating effects of a stroke are often permanent because dead brain cells cannot be replaced.

PREP KIT continued

Vital Vocabulary

acute coronary syndrome (ACS) A spectrum of clinical disease that refers to unstable angina and acute myocardial infarction (heart attack). The most common symptom is chest pain, pressure, or discomfort.

acute myocardial infarction (AMI) Death of a portion of heart muscle caused by a coronary artery occlusion; also known as a he0art attack.

alveoli Air sacs in the lungs where gas exchange takes place.

angina Chest pain felt when the heart does not receive enough oxygen.

arteries Blood vessels that carry blood away from the heart.

arterioles The smallest branches of an artery.

atria The two upper heart chambers that receive blood from the body and lungs.

brachial pulse The pulse found on the inside of the upper arm.

bronchi The two main air passages that branch out from the trachea.

capillaries Small blood vessels that connect arterioles and venules and through whose walls various substances pass into and out of the narrow spaces between tissues and then on to the cells.

cardiovascular system System composed of the heart and a complex arrangement of connected tubes (including the arteries, arterioles, capillaries, venules, and veins) that moves blood, oxygen, nutrients, carbon dioxide, and cellular waste throughout the body.

carotid artery The major artery that supplies blood to the head and brain.

carotid pulse The pulse felt on the side of the neck, over the carotid artery.

cerebellum The part of the brain that coordinates body movements.

cerebrum The largest part of the brain, containing about 75% of the brain's total volume.

coronary arteries The blood vessels that carry blood and nutrients to the heart muscle.

cyanosis A blueness of the skin due to insufficient oxygen in the blood.

defibrillator A device used to deliver a direct current shock to the heart to restore organized cardiac electrical activity.

diaphragm A dome-shaped, sheetlike muscle that separates the chest cavity from the abdomen.

dysrhythmias Heart rhythm disturbances caused by abnormal electrical signals sent out by the heart.

electrocardiogram (ECG) A measurement of the electrical impulses generated by the cardiac pacemaker cells.

epiglottis The flaplike cartilaginous structure overhanging the entrance to the trachea that prevents food from entering the trachea during swallowing.

exhalation The act of breathing out; expiration.

femoral artery The principal artery of the thigh. It can be palpated in the groin area.

femoral pulse The pulse felt on the inside of the upper thigh.

fibrinolytic drug A medication that can dissolve a clot in a cerebral or coronary artery.

glottis The opening to the trachea.

PREP KIT continued

heart The hollow muscular organ that receives blood from the veins, sends it through the lungs to be oxygenated, then pumps it to the body via the arteries.

hypoxia A dangerous condition in which the body tissues and cells do not have enough oxygen.

inhalation The drawing of air into the lungs; inspiration.

intercostal muscles Muscles between the ribs.

ischemia A lack of oxygen that deprives tissues of necessary nutrients, resulting from partial or complete blockage of blood flow; potentially reversible because permanent injury has not yet occurred.

medulla oblongata The part of the brain that is located in the brainstem and that connects the brain to the spinal cord. It controls involuntary functions, such as breathing, heart rate, and digestion.

myocardium Heart muscle.

nervous system The brain, spinal cord, and nerve branches from the central, peripheral, and autonomic nervous systems.

pacemaker cells A mass of specialized muscle fibers in the heart that regulates the electrical function of the heart.

pharynx The portion of the airway between the nasal cavity and the larynx; the throat.

plaque A substance created by materials in the blood being deposited on the arterial walls.

pulse The pressure wave that is felt with the expansion and contraction of an artery, consistent with the heartbeat.

radial pulse The pulse felt on the thumb side of the inner wrist, alongside the radius (radial bone).

respiratory arrest The cessation of breathing.

respiratory distress A condition in which respiration becomes compromised from disease, injury, choking, or drowning; results in a limited supply of air to the lungs.

respiratory system The system of organs that controls the inhalation of oxygen and the exhalation of carbon dioxide.

septum The wall separating the left and right sides of the heart.

spinal cord The cord of nerve tissue extending through the center of the spinal column.

stridor High-pitched sound during inhalation indicating an airway obstruction.

stroke A rupturing or clogging of the blood vessels that deliver oxygen-rich blood to the brain, depriving the brain of the blood and oxygen it requires.

tissue necrosis Death of tissues due to oxygen deprivation.

trachea The cartilaginous tube extending from the larynx to its division into the primary bronchi; the windpipe.

tracheal tugging Collapsing of the trachea, causing it to draw back into the neck.

veins The blood vessels that carry blood from the tissues to the heart.

venae cavae Two large veins through which blood flows into the right atrium.

ventricles The two lower chambers of the heart.

venules Very small, thin-walled blood vessels.

vertebrae The 33 bones that make up the spinal column.

Check Your Knowledge

1. Which of the following typically occurs with AMI but not with angina?

   A. The heart muscle is deprived of oxygen for only a short period.

   B. Chest pain or discomfort is not relieved by rest and/or nitroglycerin.

   C. There is a lower chance of causing permanent damage to the heart.

   D. Chest pain or discomfort is quickly relieved by rest and/or nitroglycerin.

2. The MOST common symptom(s) of angina and myocardial infarction is/are:

   A. chest pain or discomfort.

   B. sudden shortness of breath.

   C. nausea and severe anxiety.

   D. severe weakness or fatigue.

3. The heart rate of the average adult at rest is:

   A. 40 to 50 beats/min.

   B. 60 to 100 beats/min.

   C. 80 to 90 beats/min.

   D. 90 to 120 beats/min.

4. Which of the following people would MOST likely experience vague or unusual symptoms of acute myocardial infarction?

   A. 50-year-old man with a history of hypertension

   B. 70-year-old woman with a history of diabetes

   C. 62-year-old man with a history of numerous strokes

   D. 45-year-old woman who frequently abuses cocaine

5. Which of the following people is experiencing classic signs and symptoms of a stroke?

   A. 44-year-old woman with progressively worsening headaches over the past month and an irregular pulse

   B. 71-year-old man with blurred vision in both eyes, tingling in both hands, and a mild headache

   C. 60-year-old woman with progressive, generalized weakness and episodes of nausea and vomiting

   D. 52-year-old man with sudden weakness to the left side of his body, slurred speech, and facial droop

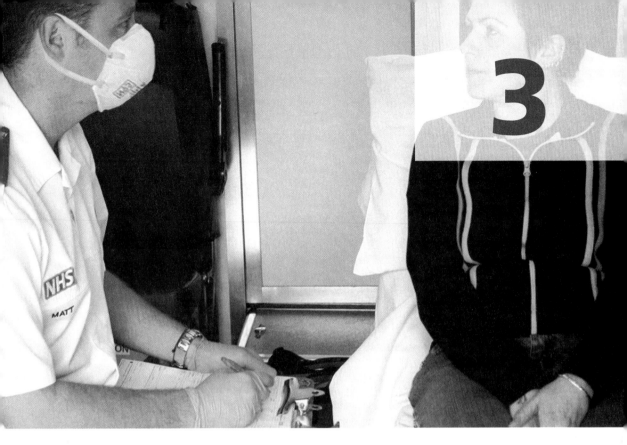

Patient Assessment

Assessing the Emergency Scene

Your first task at the scene of an emergency—whether in the hospital or in the prehospital setting—is to evaluate for hazards that could threaten the safety of those involved in providing care. You must ensure both your own personal safety and the safety of other health care providers and bystanders. Your responsibility to assess the person and provide care begins once the scene is safe **FIGURE 3-1**. If the scene is unsafe, call for the appropriate resources (eg, hospital security, fire department, law enforcement).

As you observe the scene, be aware of actual and potential threats to safety. Scene assessment can also reveal possible causes of the patient's condition—from small, hard-to-notice

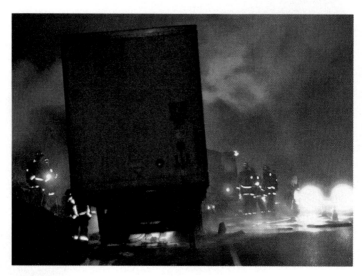

FIGURE 3-1 Assess scene safety before providing care.
© Keith D. Cullom/www.fire-image.com.

items, such as medication containers (possible medication overdose or nitroglycerin tablets or spray for a cardiac patient), to more obvious causes, such as drowning or trauma.

Emergency scenes can be chaotic. There may be distraught family members and/or bystanders. Although these people can sometimes be helpful, they can also be a hindrance. There may also be many health care providers with different levels of training. If you are the person on scene responsible for patient care, you must quickly gain control. Introduce yourself to other health care providers and bystanders in a calm, confident, and professional manner.

Assessing the Patient

Once you have sized up the scene and gained control, take standard precautions against disease transmission and begin assessing the patient. The treatment you provide to a patient is only as good as the assessment that you perform, so it is important to be thorough. A logical, systematic format, known as the primary assessment, allows you to quickly determine the most life-threatening condition the patient has. The three most important body systems in the primary assessment are the nervous system (is the patient conscious?), respiratory system (is the patient breathing?), and cardiovascular system (is the patient's heart beating? Is there uncontrolled bleeding?). This approach will help you identify situations that present immediate threats to life. Once you have assessed the patient, determine whether you have adequate personnel and equipment to provide the necessary patient care.

Assessing Responsiveness

Begin the primary assessment by checking for responsiveness (consciousness). If the patient is lying motionless, tap, gently shake their shoulder, and shout, "Are you okay?" If the patient does not respond, they are unresponsive **FIGURE 3-2**. Call for help and activate the appropriate response system, whether it is calling 9-1-1 or your hospital's code team. If help comes, have them retrieve an automated external defibrillator (AED) and proceed with your assessment. If help does not come, quickly go to get an AED and then continue caring for the patient.

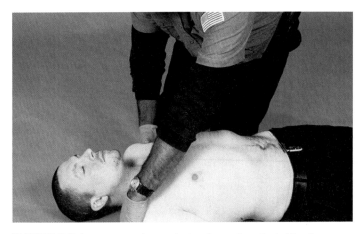

FIGURE 3-2 Assess responsiveness by tapping and gently shaking the patient's shoulder.
© Jones & Bartlett Learning. Courtesy of MIEMSS.

Assessing Breathing and Circulation

If the patient is unresponsive, check for signs of breathing and for a pulse. These two checks should occur simultaneously and take no longer than 10 seconds. Check for breathing by looking at the patient's chest to see if it is rising and falling. Normal breathing is characterized by a regular pattern of chest rise and fall. Abnormal breathing is characterized by an irregular pattern or only gasping **FIGURE 3-3**. If the patient is older than 1 year, check the pulse at the carotid artery by placing your fingers in the groove between the Adam's apple and the neck muscle on the side of the patient's neck nearest you **FIGURE 3-4**. Never try to feel the carotid pulse on both sides of the neck at the same time; doing so could block circulation to the brain. You can also check for a pulse at the femoral artery. For infants (birth to 1 year old) check the brachial pulse, located on the inside of the upper arm.

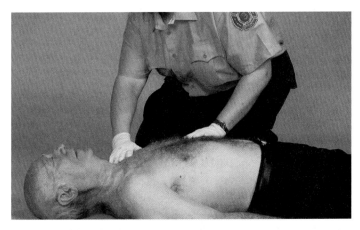

FIGURE 3-3 Check for breathing by looking at the patient's chest for movement.
© Jones & Bartlett Learning. Courtesy of MIEMSS.

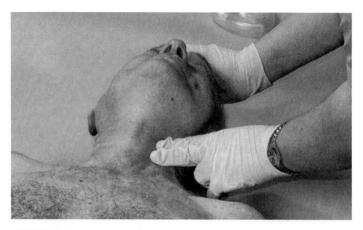

FIGURE 3-4 Check for a carotid pulse in patients older than 1 year.
© Jones & Bartlett Learning. Courtesy of MIEMSS.

Recovery Position

If the patient is unresponsive, is breathing adequately, and is not suspected of having injury to the spine, hips, or pelvis, place the patient on their side (recovery position) **FIGURE 3-5**. Monitor the patient's condition and wait for help to arrive.

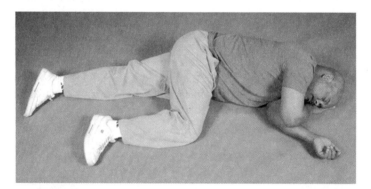

FIGURE 3-5 Recovery position for an unresponsive patient who is breathing adequately and is not suspected of having injury to the spine, hips, or pelvis.
© Jones & Bartlett Learning. Courtesy of MIEMSS.

Unresponsive, Nonbreathing Patient With a Pulse (Respiratory Arrest)

If the patient is not breathing or has abnormal breathing (ie, only gasping) but has a *definite* pulse, open the patient's airway and perform rescue breathing. For patients without a suspected spinal injury, use the head tilt–chin lift maneuver **FIGURE 3-6**. If you suspect a spinal injury, open the patient's airway with the jaw-thrust maneuver **FIGURE 3-7**. If you are unable to adequately open the patient's airway with the jaw-thrust maneuver, carefully perform the head tilt–chin lift maneuver, moving the neck only as much as is needed to open the airway. The techniques for providing rescue breathing are covered in detail in Chapter 4, *Basic Life Support for Adults and Children*.

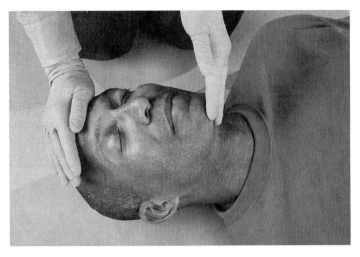

FIGURE 3-6 Open the patient's airway with the head tilt–chin lift maneuver if a neck spinal injury is not suspected.
© Jones & Bartlett Learning.

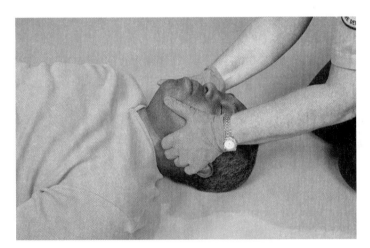

FIGURE 3-7 Use the jaw-thrust maneuver to open the patient's airway without extending the neck when a neck spinal injury is suspected.
© Jones & Bartlett Learning. Courtesy of MIEMSS.

Unresponsive, Nonbreathing Patient Without a Pulse (Cardiopulmonary Arrest)

If the patient is not breathing or has abnormal breathing (ie, only gasps) and does not have a *definite* pulse, perform 30 chest compressions, open the airway, and give 2 rescue breaths. Continue chest compressions and rescue breaths until a defibrillator (manual or automated external) has been applied and ready to analyze the patient's cardiac rhythm. The skill of cardiopulmonary resuscitation (CPR) is covered in detail in Chapter 4, *Basic Life Support for Adults and Children*. Automated external defibrillators (AEDs) are covered in Chapter 6, *Resuscitation Adjuncts*.

PREP KIT

Ready for Review

- When you arrive at an emergency scene, you must first assess the area for potential safety hazards. If the scene is unsafe, call for appropriate resources (eg, hospital security, law enforcement, fire department). Once the scene is safe take standard precautions, approach the patient, and look for possible causes of their illness or injury. Next, assess the patient as follows:
  - Check for responsiveness.
  - Check for breathing and a pulse. These two checks should be performed simultaneously and should take no more than 10 seconds.
  - If the patient is unresponsive, is breathing normally, and does not have a suspected spinal, hip, or pelvic injury, place them in the recovery position.
  - If the patient is not breathing or is breathing abnormally (ie, only gasping) but has a pulse, perform rescue breathing.
  - If the patient is not breathing or is breathing abnormally (ie, only gasping) and does not have a pulse, begin CPR (starting with chest compressions).

Vital Vocabulary

head tilt–chin lift maneuver A procedure for opening the airway in which two movements—tilting back of the forehead and lifting of the chin—are combined.

jaw-thrust maneuver A procedure for opening the airway in which the jaw is lifted and pulled forward by placing the index and middle fingers behind the mandible. This keeps the tongue from falling back into the airway; used to open the airway in patients with a suspected spinal injury.

primary assessment A step within the patient assessment process that identifies and initiates

treatment of immediate and potential life threats.

recovery position A position used to maintain a clear airway in an unresponsive patient who is breathing adequately and does not have suspected spinal, hip, or pelvic injuries.

rescue breathing A procedure in which a provider breathes for a patient who is not breathing spontaneously on their own.

unresponsive Without awareness; unconscious.

Check Your Knowledge

1. After determining that a patient is unresponsive, you should:

   A. check for breathing and for a pulse.

   B. open the airway and look in the mouth.

   C. place the patient in the recovery position.

   D. retrieve an automated external defibrillator (AED) and apply it without delay.

2. The MOST important initial action to take upon arriving at the scene of an emergency is to:

   A. call for additional assistance.

   B. determine whether any hazards exist.

   C. immediately assess the patient.

   D. obtain information from bystanders.

3. If an unresponsive patient has abnormal breathing and a pulse, you should:

    A. begin rescue breathing.

    B. place the patient on their side.

    C. start chest compressions.

    D. apply the AED without delay.

4. The recovery position should be used if a patient:

    A. is unresponsive with agonal gasps.

    B. has an injury to the spine, hips, or pelvis.

    C. is responsive with inadequate breathing.

    D. is unresponsive with adequate breathing.

5. An injured patient is unresponsive, is not breathing, and has a pulse. You are unable to open his airway with the jaw-thrust maneuver. What should you do?

    A. Attempt to perform rescue breathing.

    B. Position the patient on their side.

    C. Carefully perform the head tilt–chin lift maneuver.

    D. Begin CPR, starting with chest compressions.

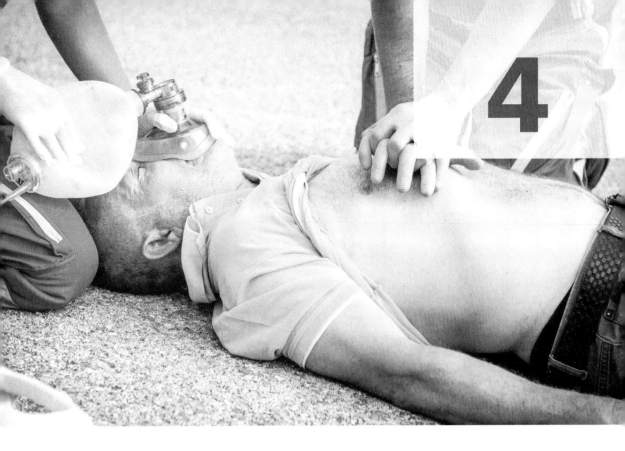

Basic Life Support for Adults and Children

Patient Assessment

As described in Chapter 3, *Patient Assessment*, your primary assessment of any motionless patient begins by assessing responsiveness. If the patient is responsive (conscious) and breathing normally, assist them as needed. However, if the patient is unresponsive (unconscious), quickly look at the patient's chest to see if it is rising and falling at a regular rate, indicating that they are breathing normally, and check for a pulse. These two checks should occur simultaneously and take no more than 10 seconds. If the patient is unresponsive but is breathing normally and has a pulse, position them in the recovery position as long as there is no suspected injury to the spine, hips, or pelvis. If the patient is unresponsive, is not breathing or is breathing abnormally (ie, only gasping), and does not have a pulse, begin cardiopulmonary resuscitation (CPR), starting with chest compressions. See page XX.

Check for Responsiveness

As previously discussed, your assessment of any motionless patient begins by assessing responsiveness. If an unresponsive patient is lying facedown, you must carefully turn them onto their back. Roll the patient, keeping the head, neck, shoulders, back, and pelvis aligned to avoid twisting the body and aggravating a spinal injury if one exists.

After the patient is properly positioned, tap them, shake their shoulders, and shout, "Are you okay?" If the patient is unresponsive, call for help. Use your cell phone, if available, to call 9-1-1 or activate the emergency response system. If bystanders are present, ask them to call for help **FIGURE 4-1**.

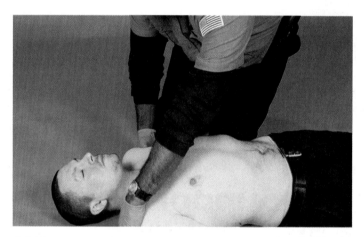

FIGURE 4-1 Determine responsiveness.
© Jones & Bartlett Learning. Courtesy of MIEMSS.

Check for Breathing and a Pulse

If the patient is unresponsive, assess for breathing by looking to see if the chest is rising and falling normally while simultaneously checking for a pulse; this assessment should take no more than 10 seconds and will determine if CPR is needed or if the patient requires only rescue breathing.

In an adult or child, the pulse is checked by locating the carotid artery at the side of the neck nearest you with your index and middle fingers. Locate the **thyroid cartilage** (Adam's apple)—the cartilaginous (firm midline) protuberance in the center of the neck—and slide your fingers toward you, into the groove at the side of the neck. Press down gently to feel for the carotid pulse. Feel for a pulse for at least 5 seconds but no more than 10 seconds **FIGURE 4-2**. You may also check for a femoral pulse, as described in Chapter 2, *Understanding the Human Body*. If a pulse is present but the patient is not breathing or is breathing abnormally (ie, only gasping), provide rescue breathing. If a pulse is absent, perform CPR starting with chest compressions. Practice by feeling your own pulse.

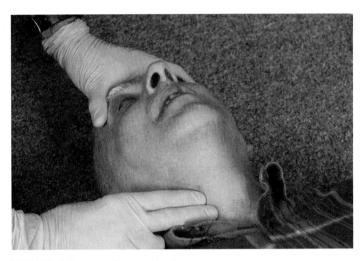

FIGURE 4-2 Palpate the carotid pulse.
© Jones & Bartlett Learning. Courtesy of MIEMSS.

Opening the Airway and Providing Rescue Breathing

If an unresponsive patient is not breathing or is breathing abnormally (ie, only gasping) but has a pulse, you will need to provide rescue breathing.

Before providing rescue breathing, you must first open the patient's airway. When a person becomes unconscious, all of the body's muscles relax, including the tongue. The relaxed tongue can fall back into the throat (pharynx) and block the airway. Because the tongue is attached to the base of the jaw, moving the jaw forward moves the tongue away from the back of the throat. In some cases, this may be all that is needed to restore breathing. There are two common maneuvers for opening the airway: the head tilt–chin lift maneuver and the jaw-thrust maneuver.

The head tilt–chin lift maneuver is used when no spinal injury is suspected. Place one hand, palm down, on the patient's forehead and tilt the head back. Place two fingers of your other hand on the bony part of the patient's chin and lift up **FIGURE 4-3**. In children, do not hyperextend the neck as you tilt the head back. In a child, neck hyperextension may cause the trachea to collapse or narrow, resulting in obstruction of the airway.

If you suspect that the patient has a spinal injury, you must open the airway in a way that protects the spinal cord. The jaw-thrust maneuver allows you to lift the patient's jaw without tilting the head back or extending the neck. Place your index and middle fingers on the angles of the lower jaw and your thumbs on the cheekbones. Move the lower jaw forward without tilting the head back **FIGURE 4-4**. If the jaw-thrust maneuver is unsuccessful, carefully perform the head tilt–chin lift maneuver—even if you suspect a spinal injury. The patient will die if their airway is not open.

Rescue breathing is the simple skill of blowing air into the lungs of a nonbreathing (apneic) patient. If a pulse is present but the patient is not breathing, you must continue to breathe for the patient. Rescue breathing rates for the child and adult are listed in TABLE 4-1.

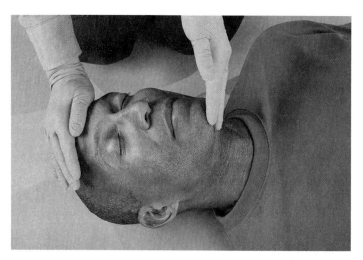

FIGURE 4-3 Place one hand on the patient's forehead and the other hand under the patient's chin. This is called the head tilt–chin lift maneuver.
© Jones & Bartlett Learning.

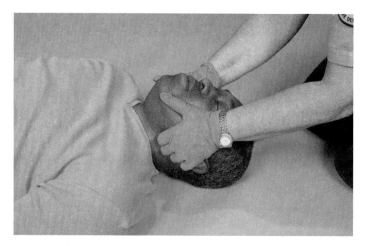

FIGURE 4-4 Opening the patient's airway with the jaw-thrust maneuver.
© Jones & Bartlett Learning. Courtesy of MIEMSS.

TABLE 4-1 Rescue Breathing Rates

Child (1 year of age to the onset of puberty [12 to 14 years of age])	One breath every 2 to 3 seconds (20 to 30 breaths per minute)
Adult (onset of puberty and older)	One breath every 6 seconds (10 breaths per minute)

© Jones & Bartlett Learning.

Deliver each rescue breath over a period of 1 second—just enough to produce visible chest rise. *Do not* ventilate too fast or with too much volume, a condition known as **hyperventilation**. Hyperventilating the patient may force more air into the stomach than the lungs (gastric distention); it may also cause increased pressure within the chest cavity and reduce blood return to the heart.

If the chest does not rise, reposition the head and attempt to deliver another breath. If two attempts at delivering rescue breathing are unsuccessful, you should suspect an airway obstruction that needs to be cleared. Management of an airway obstruction is presented later in this chapter.

Rescue breathing can be performed with various barrier ventilation devices or more advanced ventilation devices. When you respond to an emergency as part of your job, you will have the necessary ventilation equipment to prevent disease transmission. When you are not on duty, you may not have ventilation devices readily available. In this situation, you must weigh the potential good to the patient against the limited risk of contracting an infectious disease through unprotected mouth-to-mouth breathing. To eliminate this risk, you should carry a pocket rescue mask or other barrier device in case you need it when you are off duty. Detailed information about ventilation devices can be found in Chapter 6, *Resuscitation Adjuncts*.

Mouth-to-Mask Method

Follow these steps when performing mouth-to-mask rescue breathing:

1. Position yourself at the patient's head.
2. Open the patient's airway with the head tilt–chin lift or the jaw-thrust maneuver.
3. Place the mask over the patient's mouth and nose.
4. Using both hands, grasp the mask and the patient's jaw. Press down on the mask with your thumbs as you lift up on the jaw with your fingers. This will create a good seal between the mask and the face **FIGURE 4-5**.
5. Breathe into the one-way valve. Each breath should occur over a period of 1 second—ensure that it is just enough to produce visible chest rise **FIGURE 4-6**. Release pressure on the mask to allow air to escape.

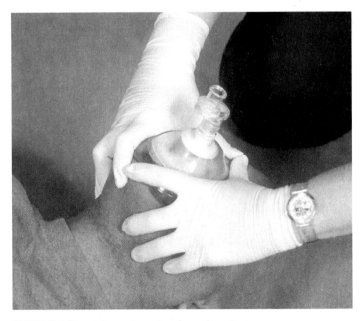

FIGURE 4-5 Seal the mask against the patient's face.
© Jones & Bartlett Learning. Courtesy of MIEMSS.

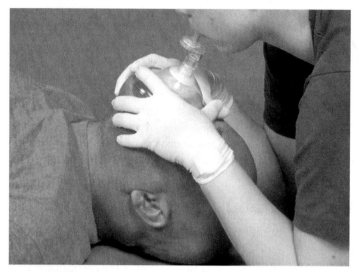

FIGURE 4-6 Place your mouth over the one-way valve and begin rescue breathing.
© Jones & Bartlett Learning. Courtesy of MIEMSS.

Mask-to-Stoma Method

A special situation involves a nonbreathing patient who has had a laryngectomy (surgical removal of the larynx). This patient no longer has a connection between the upper airway and the lungs. Instead, the patient breathes through a small, permanent opening in the front of the neck called a stoma **FIGURE 4-7**. If the patient is not breathing, you can place a small mask over the stoma and ventilate the patient. In some patients, there is still a connection between the upper airway and the stoma. When you breathe into the stoma, the patient's mouth and nose must be closed to prevent air from flowing into the upper airway.

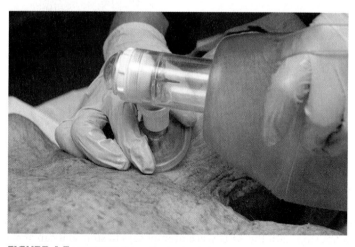

FIGURE 4-7 Ventilating through a tracheal stoma.
© Jones & Bartlett Learning. Courtesy of MIEMSS.

> **SOFT SKILL**
>
> **What Does Sudden Cardiac Arrest Look Like?**
>
> Contrary to common belief, many patients who experience sudden cardiac arrest do not suddenly become motionless. Some patients may appear to experience a seizure and their chest may continue to move—despite the fact that they are not breathing normally. This information is important to include in community CPR training programs. If the patient is not responding and is not breathing or has abnormal breathing (ie, gasping only), it should be assumed that the patient is in cardiac arrest and chest compressions should be initiated immediately.

Performing CPR

CPR is a combination of chest compressions and rescue breaths. If an unresponsive patient is not breathing or is breathing abnormally (ie, only gasping) and does not have a pulse, you must begin CPR, starting with chest compressions, until a defibrillator has been applied and is ready to analyze the patient's cardiac rhythm. CPR is also indicated if an unresponsive, nonbreathing child is pulseless or has a pulse that is fewer than 60 beats per minute with signs of poor perfusion (ie, cyanosis, decreased level of consciousness).

Adult CPR

Follow these steps to perform adult CPR:

1. Position the patient so they are flat on their back on a hard surface. Position yourself so that your knees are alongside the patient's chest.
2. Place the heel of one hand in the center of the chest, between the nipples. Place your other hand on top of the first. Lock your fingers together and pull upward so that the only thing touching the patient's chest is the heel of your hand **FIGURE 4-8**.
3. Lean forward so your shoulders are directly over your hands and the patient's sternum. Keep your arms straight and compress the sternum at least 2 inches (5 cm), using the weight of your body. The chest should not be compressed more than 2.4 inches (6 cm). Relax between compressions, allowing the chest to fully recoil; avoid leaning on the patient's chest between compressions. Give 30 compressions, counting each one out loud, at a rate of 100 to 120 per minute.
4. After 30 chest compressions, open the airway and give 2 breaths (1 second each). Ensure that each breath produces visible chest rise.
5. Continue the cycles of 30 chest compressions and 2 breaths. Do not stop unless the patient begins to move, you are replaced by someone of equal or higher training, or you are alone and become too fatigued to continue (conditions to determine when to stop are discussed later in this chapter). When the AED arrives, continue compressions while it is turned on and applied. Do not stop until the AED voice prompt says to stop so it can analyze and shock if necessary.

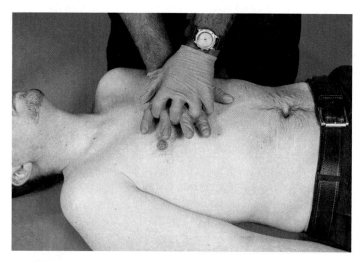

FIGURE 4-8 Performing chest compressions on an adult.
© Jones & Bartlett Learning. Courtesy of MIEMSS.

Chest Compressions

When performing chest compressions, push hard and push fast. Provide compressions at a rate of 100 to 120 per minute to a depth that is appropriate for the patient's age—at least 2 inches (5 cm) for an adult (no more than 2.4 inches [6 cm]) and at least one-third the anteroposterior depth of the chest (about 2 inches [5 cm]) for a child. Allow the chest to fully recoil after each compression and avoid leaning on the patient's chest. This technique will maximize the amount of blood returned to the heart and, ultimately, the amount of blood pumped throughout the body.

Chest compressions create blood flow to the heart through filling of the coronary arteries. Every time compressions are stopped, blood flow to the heart (and brain) drops to zero. It takes 5 to 10 effective compressions to reestablish effective blood flow to the heart after chest compressions are resumed. Avoid frequent or prolonged (greater than 10 seconds) interruptions in chest compressions, which lead to poor patient outcomes.

Chest Compression Fraction

Chest compression fraction is the total percentage of time during a resuscitation attempt in which chest compressions are being performed. Make every effort to maintain a chest compression fraction of at least 60% (the higher the better). The more frequent the interruptions in chest compressions, the lower the compression fraction will be. Low compression fractions lead to worse patient outcomes.

Child CPR

Follow these steps to perform child CPR:

1. Position the patient so they are flat on their back on a hard surface. Position yourself so that your knees are alongside the patient's chest.

2. Place the heel of one hand in the center of the chest, between the nipples **FIGURE 4-9**. For larger children, you should use two hands, as with the adult.

3. Lean forward so your shoulders are directly over your hand(s) and the patient's sternum. Keep your arms straight and compress the chest at least one-third the anteroposterior depth of the chest (about 2 inches [5 cm]). Relax between compressions, allowing the chest to fully recoil; do not lean on the chest between compressions. Give 30 compressions, counting each one out loud, at a rate of 100 to 120 per minute.

4. After 30 chest compressions, open the airway and give 2 breaths (1 second each). Ensure that each breath produces visible chest rise.

5. Continue the cycles of 30 chest compressions and 2 breaths. Do not stop unless the patient begins to move, you are replaced by someone of equal or higher training, or you are alone and become too fatigued to continue (conditions to determine when to stop are discussed later in this chapter). When the AED arrives, continue compressions while it is turned on and installed. Do not stop until the AED voice prompt tells you to "not touch the patient."

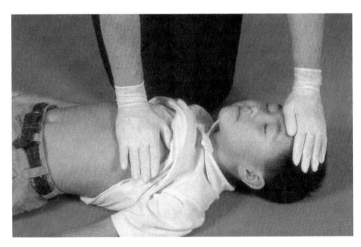

FIGURE 4-9 Performing chest compressions on a child.
© Jones & Bartlett Learning. Courtesy of MIEMSS.

Two-Person CPR

Whenever possible, two providers should work together to perform CPR. Two-person CPR has several distinct advantages over one-person CPR:

- Providers do not tire as quickly and resuscitation efforts can be more effective.
- One provider can perform chest compressions while the other provider checks the effectiveness of the compressions by monitoring for a pulse. You should be able to feel a carotid pulse during adequately performed chest compressions.

In two-person CPR, one provider performs chest compressions and the second provider delivers rescue breaths **FIGURE 4-10**. If the patient is an adult, a compression-to-ventilation ratio of 30 to 2 should be used. If the patient is a child, a compression-to-ventilation ratio of 15 to 2 should be used.

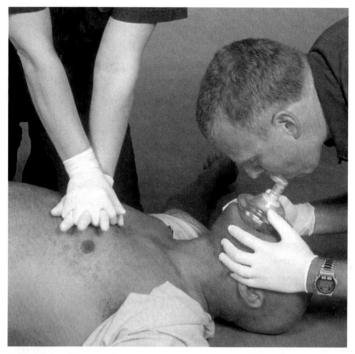

FIGURE 4-10 Performing two-person CPR.
© Jones & Bartlett Learning. Courtesy of MIEMSS.

Providers should try to work on opposite sides of the patient so they can switch functions without getting in each other's way. When two providers are performing CPR, they should switch functions every 2 minutes in order to minimize provider fatigue. Unrecognized provider fatigue can result in chest compressions that are too shallow and/or too slow. The providers should switch positions quickly so that chest compressions are not interrupted for more than 5 seconds.

When an advanced airway (ie, King LT, laryngeal mask airway, i-Gel, endotracheal tube) is in place during two-person adult or child CPR, the providers should no longer deliver cycles of CPR. Instead, they should ventilate the adult or child at a rate of 10 breaths per minute (1 breath every 6 seconds) and perform continuous chest compressions at a rate of 100 to 120 per minute. Providers should not attempt to synchronize breaths and compressions; there should be no pause in chest compressions to deliver breaths.

FYI

Asynchronous Ventilation

Depending on your local protocol, you can consider delivering 1 breath every 6 seconds (10 breaths/min) to provide asynchronous ventilation during continuous chest compressions before placement of an advanced airway.

Stopping CPR

You can discontinue CPR in the following situations:

- Return of spontaneous circulation occurs (a pulse returns) or signs of life return.
- Another trained provider replaces you.
- A physician tells you to stop.
- You are too physically exhausted to continue.
- The scene becomes unsafe.

CPR Complications and Errors

Even when CPR is performed correctly, there are potential complications, including the following:

- Fractures of the ribs or sternum
- Separation of the rib cartilage
- Bruising of the heart and lungs
- Puncture of the lungs, liver, spleen, or heart from fractured ribs
- Ruptured lungs (most often associated with excessive ventilation of the lungs in children and infants)

You can also minimize the risk of these complications by paying careful attention to your form. Do not let excitement make you careless. The following are some common mistakes people make when performing rescue breathing and CPR:

- Failing to adequately open the airway
- Failing to maintain an open airway
- Failing to maintain an adequate mask seal over the nose and mouth
- Not providing adequate breaths or breathing too fast or too forcefully
- Completing CPR cycles too slowly or too quickly
- Not placing the patient on a hard or level surface for effective chest compressions
- Performing chest compressions with the elbows bent instead of with straight arms
- Performing chest compressions with the hands in the wrong location (often too low on the sternum)
- Using the wrong compression rate
- Performing chest compressions that are too shallow or too deep or with jerky movements

---

FYI

Chest Compression Depth

An upper limit of chest compression depth has been identified for the adult. The provider should compress the chest at least 2 inches (5 cm) but no greater than 2.4 inches (6 cm). Practically speaking, it is impossible to assess such a precise depth without an audiovisual CPR monitoring device that provides immediate feedback **FIGURE 4-11**. If such a device is available, use it.

Although injuries—while not life threatening—have been reported when the chest is compressed beyond 2.4 inches (6 cm), it is more dangerous to compress too lightly than it is to compress too forcefully.

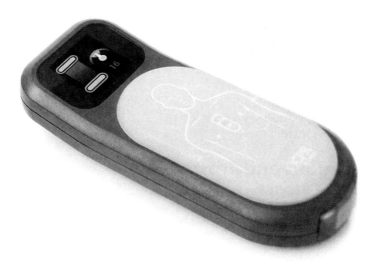

FIGURE 4-11 CPR feedback devices help ensure a consistent rate and depth of compression.
Courtesy of Laerdal Medical.

Airway Obstruction

Airway obstruction (choking) is responsible for thousands of deaths each year in the United States. According to the National Safety Council's Injury Facts 2017, choking is the fourth leading cause of unintentional injury death. Of the 5,051 people who died from choking in 2015, 2,848 were older than 74 years of age. You must be able to quickly distinguish an airway obstruction from other causes of sudden respiratory failure, such as heart attack or stroke—conditions that require different treatment. Immediate recognition and removal of the obstruction is the key to preventing hypoxia (low oxygen levels in the blood), loss of consciousness, and cardiac arrest, which will ultimately occur if the obstruction is not removed.

Causes of Airway Obstruction

Food is the most common foreign body airway obstruction in a conscious adult. Small objects, such as toys, coins, and pieces of burst balloon, are common causes of airway obstruction in children. In any unresponsive patient, the tongue is the most common cause of airway obstruction **FIGURE 4-12**.

FYI

Finger Sweeps

Do not perform blind finger sweeps in any patient—regardless of their age—as doing so may force the object farther into the airway. Attempt to remove a foreign body *only* if you can see it and easily retrieve it.

Another cause of airway obstruction is swelling of the airway passages. Swelling can result from many conditions, such as a severe allergic reaction, infections such as croup or epiglottitis, or trauma. If you are unsure whether the obstruction is caused by a foreign body or by swelling, assume the obstruction

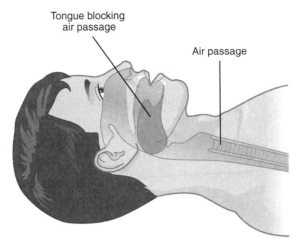

Tongue blocking
air passage

Air passage

FIGURE 4-12 The tongue is the most common cause of airway obstruction in unresponsive patients of all ages.
© Jones & Bartlett Learning.

is a foreign body. If you believe the cause of the obstruction is swelling, request advanced life support personnel immediately.

Types of Airway Obstruction

Airway obstructions are classified as being mild (partial) or severe (complete). With a mild airway obstruction, the patient has adequate air exchange. They are responsive, can cough forcefully, and may be able to speak with difficulty. If the patient is coughing, encourage them to continue, as coughing will frequently clear the obstruction. Do not interfere with the patient's own attempts to expel the obstruction; doing so may result in a severe airway obstruction. Remain with the patient and be ready to intervene if their condition deteriorates.

A severe airway obstruction occurs when the airway is completely blocked. In this case, the patient will be unable to speak, cough, cry, or breathe. The patient may display the universal distress signal for choking **FIGURE 4-13**. When the airway is severely obstructed, the skin may turn blue in lighter-skinned patients or gray in darker-skinned patients (cyanosis) and the patient may lose consciousness. Cardiac arrest will follow if the obstruction is not quickly removed.

Managing Airway Obstruction in Responsive Adults and Children

To determine whether a responsive patient has an obstructed airway, see if they are able to talk and exchange air. Ask the patient, "Are you choking?" If the patient nods yes and cannot talk, perform abdominal thrusts, also known as the Heimlich maneuver. This technique can force air from the lungs, creating an artificial cough that can expel the foreign object. If more than one provider is present, one provider should summon help while the other provider tends to the patient.

Follow these steps when performing abdominal thrusts on a responsive adult or child:

1. Stand or kneel behind the patient and wrap your arms around their waist.
2. Make a fist with one hand and place the thumb side against the abdomen, just above the umbilicus (navel) and well below the sternum (breastbone) **FIGURE 4-14**.

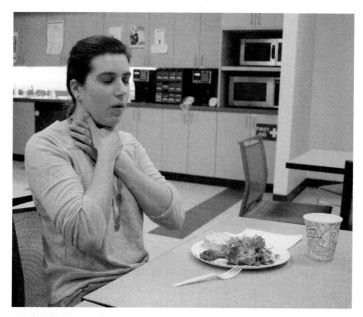

FIGURE 4-13 Universal distress signal for choking.
© Jones & Bartlett Learning.

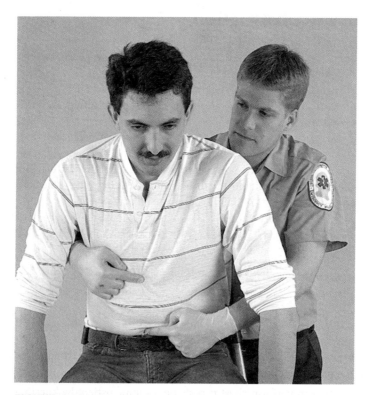

FIGURE 4-14 Locate the patient's breastbone and navel.
© Jones & Bartlett Learning. Courtesy of MIEMSS.

3. Grasp your fist with your other hand and give quick, inward and upward thrusts into the abdomen. The force of these thrusts will often be enough to relieve the obstruction **FIGURE 4-15**.

4. Continue delivering abdominal thrusts until the obstruction is relieved or the patient becomes unresponsive.

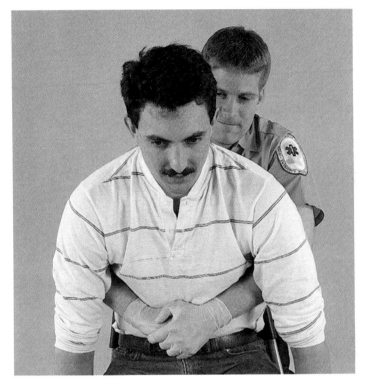

FIGURE 4-15 Give abdominal thrusts.
© Jones & Bartlett Learning. Courtesy of MIEMSS.

Special Situations

In some circumstances, you may not be able to reach around the waist of the responsive patient because they are obese or in the later stages of pregnancy. You would not want to push on the abdomen of a patient in the later stages of pregnancy. In these situations, you should perform **chest thrusts** instead of abdominal thrusts **FIGURE 4-16**.

Follow these steps to perform chest thrusts:

1. Stand behind the patient with your arms under the patient's armpits and wrap your arms around the chest.

2. Place the thumb side of one hand in the middle of the chest, between the nipples.

3. Grasp the fist with your other hand and pull inward on the chest until the obstruction is relieved or the patient becomes unresponsive.

When necessary, you can perform chest thrusts on a supine patient by kneeling close to them and delivering downward thrusts in the middle of the chest, between the nipples.

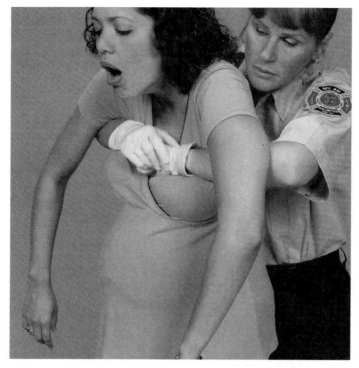

FIGURE 4-16 Give chest thrusts to an obese or pregnant patient.
© Jones & Bartlett Learning. Courtesy of MIEMSS.

Managing Airway Obstruction in Unresponsive Adults and Children

If the patient is unresponsive when you arrive at their side, begin your assessment as you would for any other unresponsive patient. However, if the adult or child becomes unresponsive during your attempts at relieving an airway obstruction, follow these steps:

1. Carefully support the patient to the ground and immediately call for help (or send someone to call for help).

2. Perform chest compressions, utilizing the same landmark as you would for CPR **FIGURE 4-17**. Perform 30 chest compressions if you are alone or if the patient is an adult; perform 15 compressions if two providers are present and the patient is a child. Note that for a choking patient who becomes unresponsive, a provider should begin chest compressions immediately after lowering the patient to the ground. Do not check for a pulse.

3. Open the airway and look in the mouth. If you see an object and can easily remove it, remove it with your fingers and attempt to ventilate. If you do not see an object, resume chest compressions.

4. Continue the sequence of performing chest compressions, opening the airway, and looking inside the mouth until the obstruction is relieved or advanced life support personnel take over.

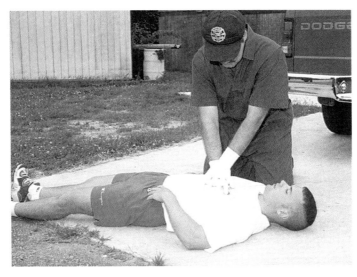

FIGURE 4-17 Perform chest compressions on an unresponsive adult or child with an airway obstruction.
© Jones & Bartlett Learning. Courtesy of MIEMSS.

After 2 minutes (about 5 cycles) of CPR, if someone has not already done so, the health care provider should go for help.

Once the obstruction is relieved and your breaths produce visible chest rise, check for a pulse. If the patient does not have a pulse, continue CPR (compressions and ventilations) until help arrives.

PREP KIT

Ready for Review

- Basic life support for adults and children follows the same general approach:
  - Determine if the patient is unresponsive, then check for breathing and a pulse; these two checks should occur simultaneously and take no longer than 10 seconds.
  - If the patient is breathing adequately, place them in the recovery position.
  - If the patient is not breathing or is breathing abnormally (ie, only gasping) but has a pulse, perform rescue breathing.
  - If a pulse is absent, begin CPR starting with chest compressions.
- Use the jaw-thrust maneuver to open the airway if you suspect a spinal injury and use the head tilt–chin lift maneuver if you do not suspect a spinal injury. In children, take care not to hyperextend the neck. If the jaw-thrust maneuver does not adequately open the airway, carefully perform a head tilt–chin lift maneuver—even if a spinal injury is suspected.
- Rescue breathing can be performed with a barrier ventilation device or more advanced devices.

- Rescue breathing should be performed at a rate of 1 breath every 6 seconds (10 breaths per minute) for adults and 1 breath every 2 to 3 seconds (20 to 30 breaths per minute) for children.
- Avoid hyperinflating the lungs (hyperventilation), as doing so may result in an increase in pressure within the chest cavity and decrease the amount of blood that returns to the heart. Hyperventilation may also result in gastric distention.
- Be sure to deliver each rescue breath over a period of 1 second—just enough to produce visible chest rise.
- If the airway is obstructed in a responsive adult or child, kneel or stand behind the patient and perform abdominal thrusts (Heimlich maneuver). Give abdominal thrusts until the obstruction is relieved or the patient becomes unresponsive.
- For an unresponsive adult or child with an airway obstruction, perform chest compressions. Move to the head, open the airway, and look in the patient's mouth. If you can see an object that can easily be removed, remove it with your fingers and attempt to ventilate. Do not perform a blind finger sweep. If you cannot see an object, resume chest compressions. Continue the sequence of performing chest compressions, opening the airway, and looking in the mouth until the obstruction is relieved or advanced life support personnel take over.
- If a patient does not have a pulse, begin CPR. CPR is a combination of chest compressions and rescue breathing.
- Chest compressions should be performed at a rate of 100 to 120 per minute. Perform 30 compressions and 2 breaths for adults and in all one-person CPR.
- Perform 15 compressions and 2 breaths for two-person infant or child CPR.
- Allow full chest recoil between compressions; do not lean on the chest. Avoid interruptions in CPR for greater than 10 seconds.
- Compress the adult's chest at least 2 inches (5 cm) but no more than 2.4 inches (6 cm).
- Compress the child's chest at least one-third the anteroposterior depth of the chest (about 2 inches [5 cm]).

Vital Vocabulary

abdominal thrusts A method of dislodging food or other foreign material from the throat of a person who is choking and responsive; also known as the *Heimlich maneuver*.

airway obstruction An airway blockage that prevents air from reaching a person's lungs.

apneic Absence of spontaneous breathing.

chest compression fraction The total percentage of time during a resuscitation attempt in which active chest compressions are being performed.

chest thrusts A maneuver used to expel objects from the throat of a person who is responsive and has an airway obstruction, particularly infants and patients who are obese or pregnant.

croup An infectious disease of the upper respiratory system that may cause airway obstruction and is characterized by a barking cough.

epiglottitis Inflammation of the epiglottis.

PREP KIT continued

Heimlich maneuver A method of dislodging food or other foreign material from the throat of a person who is choking and responsive; also known as *abdominal thrusts*.

hyperventilation Rapid or deep breathing that lowers the blood carbon dioxide level below normal

laryngectomy Surgical removal (partial or complete) of the larynx, usually due to disease of the larynx (ie, cancer).

larynx The organ of voice production; also called the *voice box*.

mild airway obstruction A condition in which the airway is partially blocked. The patient is able to exchange air in the lungs and cough forcefully but has some degree of respiratory distress.

severe airway obstruction A condition in which the airway is completely blocked and no air exchange is possible.

stoma An opening in the front of the neck through which a person breathes if their larynx has been surgically removed (laryngectomy).

thyroid cartilage The cartilaginous protuberance in the center of the neck; also referred to as the *Adam's apple*.

Check Your Knowledge

1. An unresponsive man is found lying facedown and is not moving. After moving him to his back, you should:

    A. open his airway.

    B. check for breathing and a pulse.

    C. begin CPR, starting with compressions.

    D. place him in the recovery position.

2. You attempt to open an unresponsive, injured person's airway with the jaw-thrust maneuver but are unsuccessful. You should:

    A. carefully perform a head tilt–chin lift maneuver.

    B. hyperextend the head to ensure a patent airway.

    C. quickly place the patient in the recovery position.

    D. grasp the tongue and lower jaw and carefully lift.

3. A 20-year-old man is unresponsive, is not breathing, and has a pulse. What is the appropriate rescue breathing rate for him?

    A. 6 breaths per minute

    B. 10 breaths per minute

    C. 20 breaths per minute

    D. 30 breaths per minute

4. How should you determine if an unresponsive patient is breathing?

    A. Look for cyanosis around the patient's mouth.

    B. Look, listen, and feel for air at the nose and mouth.

    C. Place your hand under the patient's nose for 10 seconds.

    D. Look at the patient's chest to see if it is rising and falling.

5. Proper treatment for a 5-year-old child who is not breathing and does not have a pulse includes:

  A. initiating CPR and sending someone to retrieve a defibrillator.

  B. ventilating the child at a rate of 20 to 30 breaths per minute.

  C. compressing the sternum to a depth of no greater than 1 inch (3 cm).

  D. providing chest compressions at a rate of at least 80 per minute.

6. When is it appropriate to perform chest compressions on a patient who has a pulse?

  A. An adult patient does not respond to rescue breathing.

  B. A child has a heart rate of less than 60 beats per minute and signs of poor perfusion.

  C. An adult patient has an airway obstruction and is coughing forcefully.

  D. A responsive child has difficulty breathing and a rapid, weak pulse.

7. Which of the following statements regarding chest compressions is correct?

  A. Compress the adult's chest to a depth of at least 2 inches (5 cm).

  B. In most children, the chest is compressed to a depth of 1 inch (3 cm).

  C. Use the heel of one hand when compressing the chest of a large child.

  D. Chest compressions should be performed on a person who is choking and responsive.

8. When an advanced airway device has been inserted into a patient during two-person CPR, you should:

  A. deliver a ventilation rate of 20 breaths/min.

  B. deliver each breath over a period of 2 to 3 seconds.

  C. avoid pausing compressions to deliver rescue breaths.

  D. deliver compressions at a rate of at least 80 per minute.

9. A 60-year-old woman becomes unconscious while you are treating her for a severe airway obstruction. After carefully lowering her to the ground, you should:

  A. check for a carotid pulse.

  B. attempt to ventilate her.

  C. perform a finger sweep.

  D. perform chest compressions.

10. A patient with a mild airway obstruction:

  A. should be treated with abdominal thrusts.

  B. moves some air and may be able to speak.

  C. should be highly discouraged from coughing.

  D. often becomes cyanotic and unresponsive.

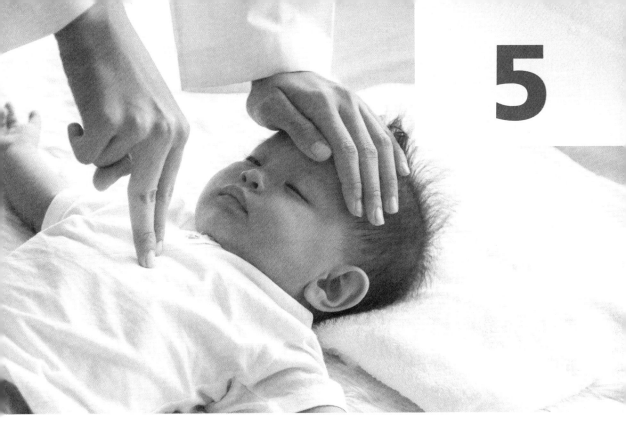

5

Basic Life Support for Infants

Assessment of an Infant

Cardiac arrest in infants (younger than 1 year), as in children, usually results from respiratory failure. Other causes may include injury, suffocation, airway obstruction, smoke inhalation, infection, drowning, or sudden unexplained infant death (SUID). In these situations, the heart is deprived of necessary oxygen and subsequently fails. TABLE 5-1 describes common issues that affect children and infants.

The primary assessment of a motionless infant is almost the same as it is for an adult or a child; a few of the actual skills are different. Begin by checking responsiveness. If the infant is responsive, assist them if needed. If the infant is unresponsive, however, quickly look at the patient's chest to see if it is rising and falling, indicating that they are breathing, and check for a

TABLE 5-1 Common Issues in Children and Infants

Airway Obstruction

Mild airway obstruction:
- Good air exchange
- Child or infant is responsive
- Forceful cough

Treatment: Allow position of comfort, assist young child to sit up (may sit on parent's lap); do not lay the child or infant down.

Severe airway obstruction:
- No crying or speaking
- Minimal or no air exchange
  - Cough is ineffective or absent
  - Increased breathing difficulty
  - High-pitched inhalation sound (stridor) or no noise at all
- Possible cyanosis (turning blue or gray)
- Child or infant becomes unresponsive

Treatment: Clear airway using the appropriate technique and attempt rescue breathing.

Sudden Unexplained Infant Death (SUID)

Signs and symptoms:
- Sudden death in the first year of life
- No obvious cause of death prior to investigation (unexplained)
- Baby is most commonly discovered in the early morning

First aid:
- Assess the ABCs (airway, breathing, circulation).
- Attempt to comfort the parents.
- Try to resuscitate the baby unless obvious signs of death are present (ie, rigor mortis, dependent lividity).
- Parents will be in agony from emotional distress, remorse, and guilt; avoid any comments that might suggest blame.

Child Abuse

Any child who is suspected of being abused should receive a thorough and proper medical evaluation. The case should be reported to the appropriate authorities.

Physical abuse and neglect are two forms of **child abuse**:
- Abuse: improper or excessive action resulting in injury or harm
- Neglect: failure to give sufficient attention or respect to someone who has a claim to that attention

Signs and symptoms of abuse:
- Multiple bruises in various stages of healing
- Patterns of injury (eg, cigarette burns, whip marks, handprints)
- Fresh burns, such as scalding, untreated burns, or appearance that a body part was submerged in hot liquid
- Parents seem inappropriately unconcerned
- Conflicting explanations of injury

Signs and symptoms of neglect:
- Lack of adult supervision
- Malnourished-appearing child
- Unsafe living environment
- Untreated soft-tissue injuries

State law requires that you:
- Report what you see and what you hear.
- Do not comment on what you think.
- Do not accuse parents or guardians.

pulse. These two checks should occur simultaneously and take no more than 10 seconds. If the infant is unresponsive and is breathing normally, monitor their condition until help arrives. If the infant is not breathing or is breathing abnormally (ie, only gasping) but has a pulse, provide rescue breathing. If both pulse and breathing are absent, begin cardiopulmonary resuscitation (CPR), starting with chest compressions. If bystanders are present, ask them to call for help. If there are no bystanders, provide 2 minutes of care and then use your cell phone, if available, to call 9-1-1 or activate the emergency response system.

Check for Responsiveness

When presented with a motionless infant, gently tap the infant and shout. You can also flick the soles of the infant's feet with your fingers. If the unresponsive infant is lying facedown, you must turn them onto their back. If you are alone and without a cell phone, you should complete your assessment and provide 2 minutes of care before going for help. If two health care providers are present, one should go for help as the other cares for the infant.

Check for Breathing and a Pulse

If the infant is unresponsive, assess for breathing by looking for the rising and falling of the chest while simultaneously checking for a pulse; this assessment should take no more than 10 seconds and will determine if CPR is needed or if the infant requires only rescue breathing.

Feeling the carotid pulse in an infant is difficult because infants have short necks. Therefore, you should feel for a brachial pulse, which is found on the inside of the upper arm **FIGURE 5-1**. Place your index and middle fingers on the inside of the arm and press gently to feel for a pulse. Feel for at least 5 seconds but no more than 10 seconds. If a *definite* pulse is present, provide rescue breathing. If the pulse is absent or if the pulse rate is less than 60 beats per minute with signs of poor perfusion (ie, cyanosis, pallor, decreased level of consciousness), begin CPR starting with chest compressions. Infant CPR will be discussed later in this chapter.

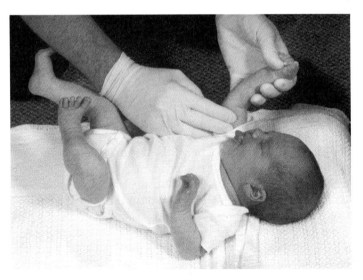

FIGURE 5-1 Check the infant's brachial pulse.
© Jones & Bartlett Learning. Courtesy of MIEMSS.

Opening the Airway and Providing Rescue Breathing

If an unresponsive infant is not breathing or is breathing abnormally (ie, only gasping) but has a pulse, you will need to provide rescue breathing (as discussed in Chapter 4, *Basic Life Support for Adults and Children*).

Before providing rescue breathing, you must first open the infant's airway. Use the head tilt–chin lift maneuver unless you suspect a spinal injury. Because infants have a proportionately large head, specifically the back of their head, it may be necessary to place padding beneath the shoulders to facilitate opening the airway. Gently tilt the infant's head. The infant's head should be tilted back less than a child's. Be careful not to hyperextend the head and neck, which can collapse or close the trachea. To lift the chin, place your finger(s) just under it, on the bony part of the jaw. Do not press on the soft tissue under the infant's chin because doing so can interfere with opening the airway **FIGURE 5-2**. If you suspect a spinal injury, open the airway with the jaw-thrust maneuver. As with the adult and child, if the jaw-thrust maneuver does not adequately open the airway, *carefully* perform the head tilt–chin lift maneuver. Simply opening the airway may restore adequate breathing.

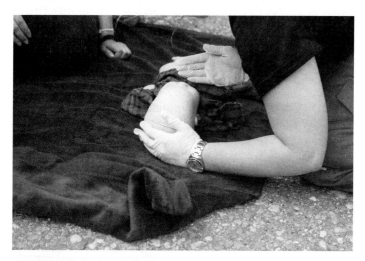

FIGURE 5-2 Open an infant's airway with the head tilt–chin lift maneuver.
© wellphoto/Shutterstock.

After opening the infant's airway, create a tight seal over the infant's mouth and nose with a ventilation mask or other barrier device. Like those needed for an adult or child, rescue breaths for an infant require only the amount of air to produce visible chest rise. In the infant, this volume can usually be accomplished by providing ventilations with the amount of air that is in your mouth. As you gently blow into the infant's mouth and nose, watch for the chest to rise and fall.

Because infants normally breathe faster than adults do, you should provide rescue breathing at a rate of 20 to 30 breaths per minute (1 breath every 2 to 3 seconds). Do not overinflate the infant's lungs by breathing too forcefully or too fast (hyperventilation). Hyperventilation can result in several negative effects; it may damage the infant's lungs, result in vomiting, distend the abdomen and make it difficult for the lungs to fully inflate, and decrease the amount of blood that returns to the heart. You can avoid these issues by maintaining an open airway and giving small puffs (1 second each)—just enough to produce visible chest rise.

If the chest does not rise, reposition the head and attempt to deliver another breath. If two attempts at delivering rescue breathing are unsuccessful, suspect an airway obstruction that needs to be cleared. Treatment for an airway obstruction is presented later in this chapter.

CPR for Infants

CPR (chest compressions and rescue breaths) is indicated for an infant if they are pulseless or if their heart rate is less than 60 beats per minute with signs of poor perfusion (ie, cyanosis, pallor, decreased level of consciousness).

CPR for infants differs from CPR for adults and children because of the infant's size. Compressions are performed with the index and middle fingers of one hand, placed on the sternum one finger width below the nipple line **FIGURE 5-3**.

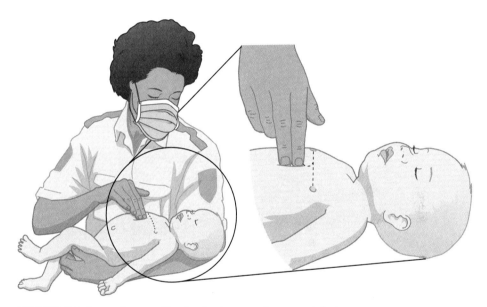

FIGURE 5-3 Correct finger position for chest compressions on an infant.
© Jones & Bartlett Learning.

With your fingers in the correct location, compress the chest with the pads of your fingertips. Compress the chest at least one-third the anteroposterior depth of the chest (about 1.5 inches [4 cm]) at a rate of 100 to 120 compressions per minute. Ensure that the chest fully recoils following each compression. After 30 chest compressions, open the airway and deliver 2 rescue breaths.

If there are bystanders, have them call for help and retrieve an AED. If you are alone and without a cell phone, give 30 compressions and 2 breaths per cycle. Perform 2 minutes of CPR and then go for help. If two health care providers are present, give 15 compressions and 2 breaths per cycle. As with adult and child CPR, two providers should switch roles every 2 minutes to minimize fatigue. Continue CPR unless the infant begins to move, you are replaced by someone of equal or higher training, or you are alone and become too fatigued to continue. When the AED arrives, continue compressions while it is turned on and applied. Do not stop until the voice prompts you to stop so it can analyze and shock if necessary. Limit interruptions in chest compressions to 10 seconds or less.

When an advanced airway (eg, laryngeal mask airway, endotracheal tube) is in place during two-person infant CPR, the providers should no longer deliver cycles of CPR. Instead, ventilate the infant at a rate of 10 breaths per minute (1 breath every 6 seconds) and perform compressions at a rate of 100 to 120 per minute. Do not attempt to synchronize breaths and compressions; there should be no pause in chest compressions to deliver breaths.

FYI

Two-Thumb Encircling Hands Technique

When two providers are performing CPR on an infant or if the patient is a **neonate** (younger than 1 month), the two-thumb encircling hands technique should be used **FIGURE 5-4**. This method has been shown to provide better blood flow than the two-finger method and is less tiresome for the provider performing compressions. Compressions should be delivered over the lower third of the sternum.

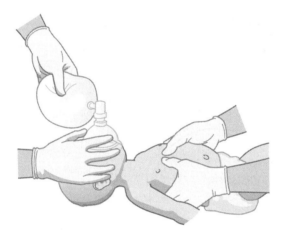

FIGURE 5-4 The two-thumb encircling hands technique is the recommended method of performing chest compressions when two providers are performing CPR on an infant or when the patient is a neonate.
© Jones & Bartlett Learning.

Airway Obstruction

Managing the Responsive Infant With an Airway Obstruction

Like children, infants also choke on food, such as grapes and nuts, and small objects, such as toys, coins, and pieces of burst balloon. An infant who exhibits signs of choking or one who is coughing may have an airway obstruction. If the infant is coughing forcefully, has adequate air exchange, and has normal skin color, suspect a mild airway obstruction. Closely observe the infant, but do not interfere with their own attempts to expel the obstruction. If the infant cannot cough, cry, or breathe, is coughing weakly, is turning blue or gray (cyanosis), or is making high-pitched sounds during inhalation (stridor), they have a severe airway obstruction and requires immediate treatment.

Follow these steps to perform care for a responsive infant with a severe airway obstruction:

1. Position the infant facedown over your forearm with their head lower than the chest. Support the infant's jaw with your hand.

2. Lower the infant and your forearm to your thigh.

3. Use the heel of your hand to give the infant five back blows (also called back slaps) between the shoulder blades **FIGURE 5-5**. Deliver each back blow with enough force to dislodge the obstruction.

4. Place the infant between your hands and arms and turn the infant face up.

5. If the back blows did not dislodge the foreign body, give five chest compressions in the same location as you do for chest compressions during cardiac arrest **FIGURE 5-6**.

6. Observe the infant throughout the process to see whether the obstruction has been dislodged. If it has not, continue the cycles of five back blows and five chest compressions until the obstruction is dislodged or the infant becomes unresponsive.

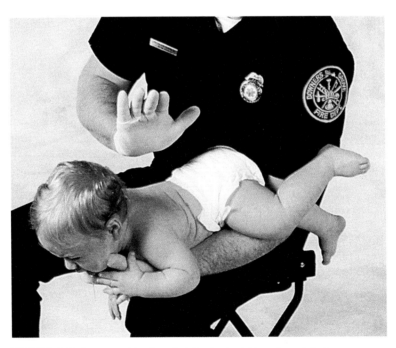

FIGURE 5-5 Correct position for administering back blows to an infant.
© Jones & Bartlett Learning. Courtesy of MIEMSS.

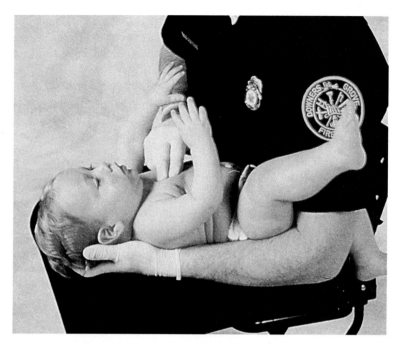

FIGURE 5-6 Finger position for chest compressions on an infant.
© Jones & Bartlett Learning. Courtesy of MIEMSS.

Managing the Unresponsive Infant With an Airway Obstruction

If the infant is unresponsive when you arrive at their side, begin your assessment as you would for any other unresponsive infant. However, if the infant becomes unresponsive during your attempts at relieving an airway obstruction, follow these steps:

1. Position the infant on a firm, flat surface and immediately call for help (or send someone to call for help).

2. Perform chest compressions, using the same landmark as you would for CPR **FIGURE 5-7**. Perform 30 chest compressions if you are alone; perform 15 compressions if 2 providers are present. As with a child or an adult, do not check for a pulse before beginning chest compressions on a choking infant who becomes unresponsive.

3. Open the airway and look in the mouth **FIGURE 5-8**. If you see an object and can easily remove it, try to remove it with your finger and attempt to ventilate. If you do not see an object, resume chest compressions.

4. Continue the sequence of performing chest compressions, opening the airway, and looking in the mouth until the obstruction is relieved or advanced life support personnel take over.

After 2 minutes (about 5 cycles) of CPR, if someone has not already done so, the health care provider should go for help.

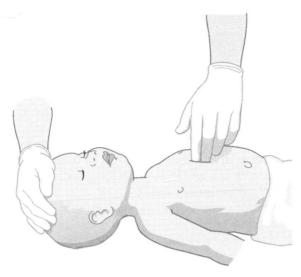

FIGURE 5-7 Perform chest compressions on an unresponsive infant with an airway obstruction.
© Jones & Bartlett Learning.

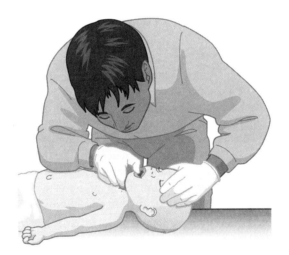

FIGURE 5-8 Check the infant's mouth for foreign object(s).
© Jones & Bartlett Learning.

Once the obstruction is relieved and your breaths produce visible chest rise, check for a pulse. If the patient has a pulse but is not breathing or is breathing abnormally (ie, only gasping), continue rescue breathing. If the patient does not have a pulse (or a pulse less than 60 beats per minute with signs of poor perfusion), continue CPR (compressions and ventilations) until help arrives.

PREP KIT

Ready for Review

- Basic life support for infants is similar to that provided for adults and children. The techniques may differ somewhat, but the same general steps apply. Check responsiveness and call for help.
  - If the infant is responsive, monitor their condition until help arrives.
  - If the infant is unresponsive, simultaneously check for breathing and a pulse; these two checks should take no more than 10 seconds. If the infant is breathing adequately, monitor their condition until help arrives.
  - If the infant is not breathing or is breathing abnormally (ie, only gasping) but has a pulse, provide rescue breathing.
  - If both pulse and breathing are absent, begin CPR starting with chest compressions.
- Use the jaw-thrust maneuver to open the airway if you suspect a spinal injury and the head tilt–chin lift maneuver if you do not suspect a spinal injury. In infants, take care not to hyperextend the neck. If the jaw-thrust maneuver does not adequately open the airway, carefully perform a head tilt–chin lift maneuver—even if a spinal injury is suspected.
- Check for a pulse at the brachial artery. If a pulse is present but the infant is not breathing or is breathing abnormally (ie, only gasping), perform rescue breathing at a rate of 20 to 30 breaths per minute (1 breath every 2 to 3 seconds). Deliver each breath over 1 second and observe for visible chest rise. Do not hyperventilate the infant, as doing so can cause gastric distention and decreased blood return to the heart.
- If there is no pulse or if the pulse rate is less than 60 beats per minute with poor perfusion, begin CPR starting with chest compressions.
  - If you are alone, use 2 fingers to compress the chest 30 times, at a rate of 100 to 120 compressions per minute, to a depth that is at least one-third the anteroposterior depth of the chest (about 1.5 inches [4 cm]). After 30 compressions, give 2 breaths.
  - If 2 providers are present or if the patient is a neonate, use the 2-thumb encircling hands technique and provide 15 compressions to 2 breaths. Compress the chest over the lower third of the sternum. Continue CPR until the infant starts to move or a defibrillator advises you to stop so it can analyze the cardiac rhythm and administer a shock if necessary .
- If the airway is obstructed in a responsive infant, perform back blows and chest thrusts until the obstruction is relieved or the infant becomes unresponsive. For an unresponsive infant with an airway obstruction, perform chest compressions. Move to the head, open the airway, and look in the patient's mouth. If you can see an object that can easily be removed, remove it with your finger and attempt to ventilate. If you cannot see an object, resume chest compressions. Continue the sequence of performing chest compressions, opening the airway, and looking in the mouth until the obstruction is relieved or advanced life support personnel take over.

PREP KIT continued

Vital Vocabulary

child abuse Any improper or excessive action that injures or otherwise harms a child or infant—includes neglect and physical, sexual, and emotional abuse.

neonate Person who is birth to 1 month of age.

sudden unexplained infant death (SUID) Death of an infant (younger than 1 year) that remains unexplained after a complete autopsy and assessment of the scene.

Check Your Knowledge

1. After determining that an infant is unresponsive, you should call for help and then:

   A. open the airway and attempt to ventilate twice.

   B. check for breathing and a pulse for up to 10 seconds.

   C. perform CPR for 2 minutes and then reassess the infant.

   D. carefully look in the mouth for a foreign body.

2. If you are alone with an infant who is unresponsive, apneic, and pulseless, you should:

   A. perform CPR for 2 minutes and go get help.

   B. immediately get help and return to the infant.

   C. perform compressions until help arrives.

   D. perform cycles of 15 compressions and 2 breaths.

3. In which of the following situations should you perform CPR on an infant?

   A. Slow breathing, brachial pulse rate of 100 beats per minute, and pink skin

   B. Not breathing, brachial pulse rate of 90 beats per minute, and cyanosis

   C. Slow breathing, brachial pulse rate of 80 beats per minute, and pallor

   D. Not breathing, brachial pulse rate of 50 beats per minute, and cyanosis

4. During two-person infant CPR, chest compressions should be performed:

   A. by compressing the chest no deeper than 0.5 to 1 inch (1 to 3 cm).

   B. by allowing partial recoil of the chest in between compressions.

   C. with two fingers over the sternum, just below the nipple line.

   D. with two thumbs and the hands encircling the infant's chest.

5. While treating a responsive infant with a severe airway obstruction, he or she becomes unresponsive. You should:

    A. check for a brachial pulse and begin CPR if the pulse is absent.

    B. continue back blows and chest thrusts until additional help arrives.

    C. place the infant on a firm, flat surface and perform chest compressions.

    D. open the infant's airway, look inside the mouth, and attempt to ventilate.

6. Which of the following statements regarding rescue breathing in the infant is correct?

    A. Deliver one breath every 2 to 3 seconds; each breath should produce visible chest rise.

    B. A rescue breathing rate of one breath every 6 seconds should be used on infants.

    C. Deliver rescue breaths at a rate of 10 breaths per minute; watch for the chest to rise.

    D. Breathing into the infant's mouth and nose may cause lung damage and should be avoided.

7. When you begin one-person CPR on an infant, you should continue until:

    A. the infant has not responded after 10 cycles of adequate CPR.

    B. the defibrillator arrives, has been applied, and begins analyzing.

    C. an EMT or a paramedic arrives and pronounces the infant dead.

    D. the infant's heart rate exceeds 40 beats per minute, even if cyanosis is present.

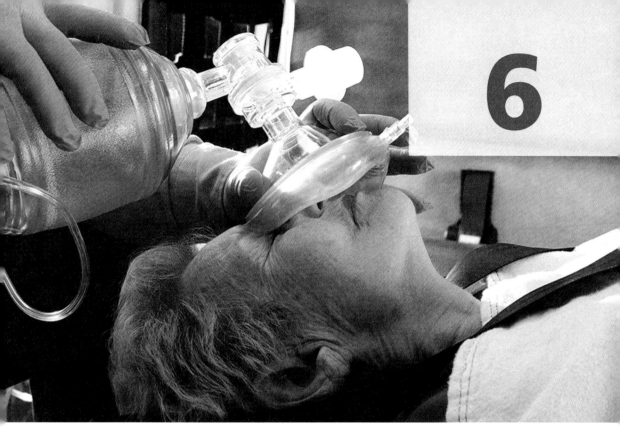

Resuscitation Adjuncts

Resuscitation Adjuncts

Successfully managing respiratory and cardiac emergencies requires quick thinking, sound skills, teamwork, and familiarity with how your equipment works. When correctly used, suction units help clear the airway, airway devices help maintain a patent (open) airway, ventilation devices provide effective barriers against disease transmission, and defibrillators enhance survival for patients experiencing cardiac arrest caused by ventricular fibrillation (VF).

Suction Units

Patients who have vomited, who have inhaled fluid or debris, or who are bleeding from the nose or mouth are in danger of an airway obstruction. You cannot maintain a patent airway or begin rescue breathing until the airway is clear and effective air exchange can occur. Suction devices can help you remove blood and other secretions from the airway, thus preventing aspiration, when vomitus, fluids, secretions, or other foreign material is inhaled into the trachea and lungs. There are two primary types of suction devices: manual devices and mechanical devices.

Manual Suction Devices

Manual suction devices that do not require batteries or an electrical source are among the most convenient to operate. These devices are always ready to work and require minimal servicing. Suction is applied by inserting the tip of the device into the patient's mouth and squeezing its handle to create a vacuum that withdraws debris **FIGURE 6-1**. Manual and mechanical suction—described in detail in the following section—are used in the same way; the only difference is the power source.

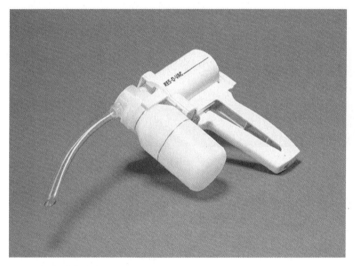

FIGURE 6-1 Manual suction device.
© Jones & Bartlett Learning. Courtesy of MIEMSS.

Mechanical Suction Devices

Mechanical suction units are powered by either rechargeable batteries or pressurized oxygen to generate a vacuum. These units require familiarity with the mechanisms for their use as well as regular maintenance and service checks **FIGURE 6-2**. Like manual suction devices, these mechanical devices also create a vacuum that draws obstructing materials from the patient's airway. To use these devices effectively, you must learn how they operate and how to control the force of the suction.

All mechanical suction devices consist of a power unit, disposable suction catheters of various sizes and shapes, an unbreakable collection bottle, suction tubing, and a supply of water for flushing out the tubing and suction catheters. Two types of suction catheters are commonly used with mechanical suction devices: the rigid-tip catheter **FIGURE 6-3** and the flexible catheter **FIGURE 6-4**.

Follow these steps when suctioning:

1. Turn the patient's head to the side. If you suspect a spinal injury, roll the patient onto their side and keep the neck and body from twisting.

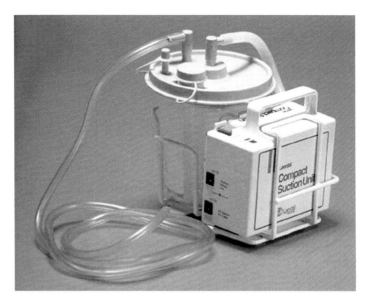

FIGURE 6-2 Battery-powered mechanical suction device.
© Jones & Bartlett Learning. Courtesy of MIEMSS.

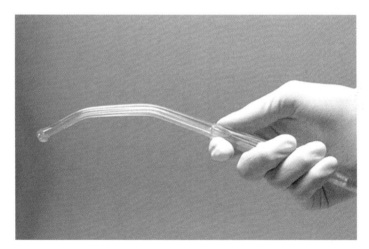

FIGURE 6-3 Rigid-tip suction catheter.
© Jones & Bartlett Learning. Courtesy of MIEMSS.

2. Open the patient's mouth and wipe away any large debris with your gloved fingers.

3. Measure the suction catheter from the corner of the patient's mouth to the earlobe. This gives you the proper depth to insert the end of the suction tip. Inserting the catheter too deeply and attempting to suction is likely to stimulate the patient's vomiting (gag) reflex.

4. Turn on the suction device, insert the suction tip, and suction as you slowly withdraw the catheter from the mouth.

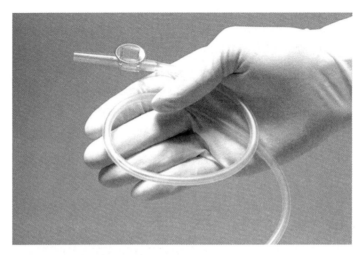

FIGURE 6-4 Flexible suction catheter.
© Jones & Bartlett Learning. Courtesy of MIEMSS.

Simple Airway Adjuncts

Once a patient's airway is clear, maintaining the open airway is extremely important. Because the tongue is the most common cause of airway obstruction in an unconscious patient, artificial airways can be used to prevent the tongue from causing a blockage. There are two types of simple airway adjuncts: oral airways and nasal airways.

Oral Airways

The most commonly used simple airway adjunct is the oropharyngeal (oral) airway **FIGURE 6-5**. It is inserted into the mouth, past the curvature of the tongue, and comes to rest in the back of the throat. This

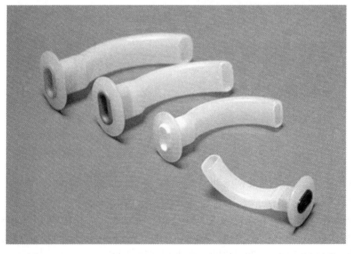

FIGURE 6-5 Oral airways.
© Jones & Bartlett Learning. Courtesy of MIEMSS.

position keeps the tongue from falling back into the throat and obstructing the airway. Improper placement could force the tongue farther into the pharynx, resulting in an airway obstruction. Because the oral airway will likely stimulate the oropharynx and cause gagging, it should be used only in unconscious patients who do not have a gag reflex.

There are various sizes of oral airways for infants, children, and adults. Selecting the correct size is important. If the oral airway is too large, it can trigger the gag reflex, and vomit could possibly be aspirated into the trachea and lungs. If the oral airway is too small, it could become an airway obstruction itself.

Follow these steps when inserting an oral airway:

1. Choose the correct size. Measure the device from the corner of the patient's mouth to the earlobe **FIGURE 6-6**. Alternatively, you can measure from the corner of the mouth to the angle of the jaw.

2. Open the patient's airway using either the head tilt–chin lift or the jaw-thrust maneuver.

3. Use a tongue depressor to depress the tongue, ensuring the tongue remains forward. Insert the oral airway sideways from the corner of the mouth, until the flange reaches the teeth **FIGURE 6-7**. Rotate the oral airway at a 90° angle and gently exert backward pressure **FIGURE 6-8** until the flange rests securely in place against the lips **FIGURE 6-9**.

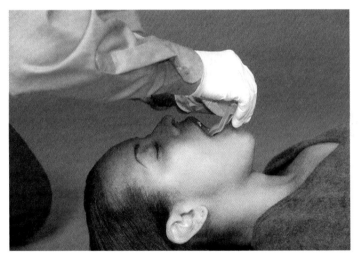

FIGURE 6-6 Proper sizing of an oral airway.
© Jones & Bartlett Learning.

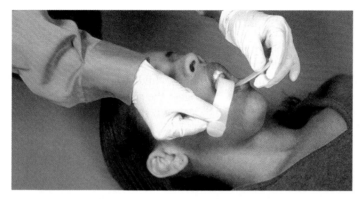

FIGURE 6-7 Insert the oral airway sideways into the corner of the mouth.
© Jones & Bartlett Learning.

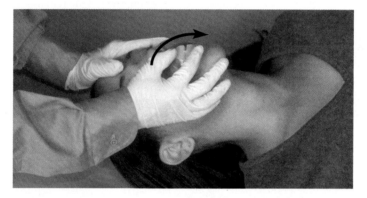

FIGURE 6-8 Rotate the oral airway at a 90° angle and exert gentle downward pressure.
© Jones & Bartlett Learning.

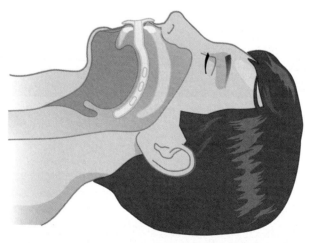

FIGURE 6-9 Interior view of the proper position of the oral airway after insertion.
© Jones & Bartlett Learning.

Nasal Airways

A semiconscious or conscious patient who has a gag reflex can usually tolerate a nasopharyngeal (nasal) airway better than an oral airway. Unlike an oral airway, the nasal airway is less likely to cause the patient to gag. It can be used on either conscious or unconscious patients, but it should not be used on patients with suspected fractures of the skull, nose, or midface.

Nasal airways are hollow devices made of soft rubber or latex. They are inserted through one of the nostrils and follow the nasal passage **FIGURE 6-10**. Bleeding is a complication that can occur when a nasal airway is inserted. As with the oral airway, choosing the correct size of nasal airway is very important. If it is too large, it will not fit into the nostril. If it is too small, it will not keep the airway open or allow adequate air exchange.

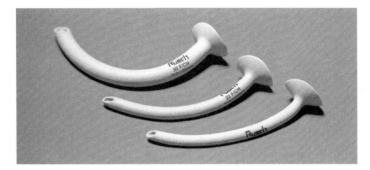

FIGURE 6-10 Nasal airways.
© Jones & Bartlett Learning. Courtesy of MIEMSS.

Follow these steps when inserting a nasal airway:

1. Choose the right size of airway. It must fit in the patient's nostril. Measure the airway from the tip of the nose to the earlobe **FIGURE 6-11**. Alternatively, you can measure from the tip of the nose to the angle of the jaw.

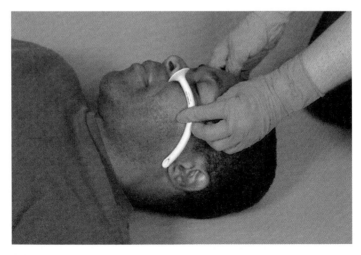

FIGURE 6-11 Proper sizing of a nasal airway.
© Jones & Bartlett Learning. Courtesy of MIEMSS.

2. Open the patient's airway using either the head tilt–chin lift or the jaw-thrust maneuver.

3. Lubricate the airway with a sterile, water-based lubricant or with sterile water or saline solution if no lubricant is available. If using the right nostril, the bevel should face the **septum**—the wall that separates the left and right nasal passages. If using the left nostril, insert the airway pointing upward, which will allow the bevel to face the septum.

4. Insert the airway through the nostril, following the nasal passage straight back, not upward **FIGURE 6-12**. **FIGURE 6-13** shows an exterior view of proper placement. **FIGURE 6-14** shows an interior view of proper placement. Do not force the airway if you meet resistance. Instead, remove the airway and try inserting it into the other nostril.

5. Listen and feel for airflow through the airway.

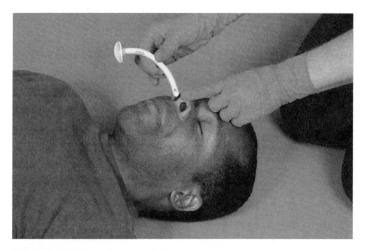

FIGURE 6-12 Inserting a nasal airway.
© Jones & Bartlett Learning. Courtesy of MIEMSS.

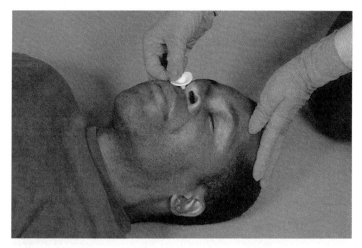

FIGURE 6-13 Exterior view of the proper position of the flange after insertion.
© Jones & Bartlett Learning.

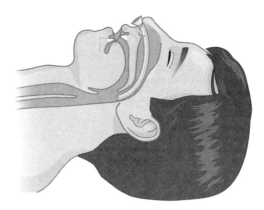

FIGURE 6-14 Interior view of the proper position of the nasal airway after insertion.
© Jones & Bartlett Learning.

Ventilation Devices

Ventilation Masks

Mouth-to-mask (or other barrier device) ventilation can deliver an adequate volume of air to a patient if the health care provider ensures a tight mask seal on the face. Ventilation masks, in general, offer some protection from disease transmission **FIGURE 6-15**. Certain types of masks have an inlet that allows oxygen tubing to be attached to the mask **FIGURE 6-16**. No matter which mask you select, you must consider a number of issues. The mask must fit well, have a one-way valve, be made of transparent material, and be available in infant, child, and adult sizes **FIGURE 6-17**. A simple barrier device, such as a face shield, may also be used, although there is no oxygen port.

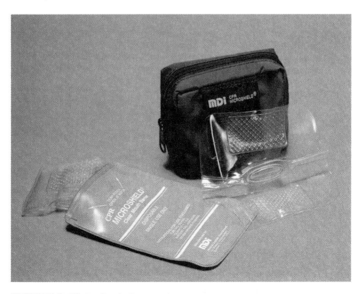

FIGURE 6-15 Barrier devices.
© Jones & Bartlett Learning. Courtesy of MIEMSS.

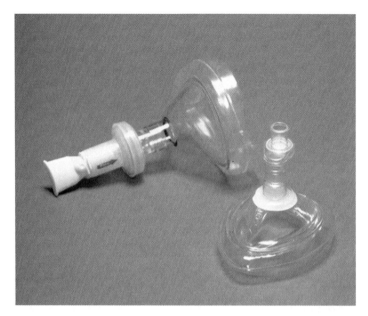

FIGURE 6-16 Types of mouth-to-mask ventilation devices.
© Jones & Bartlett Learning. Courtesy of MIEMSS.

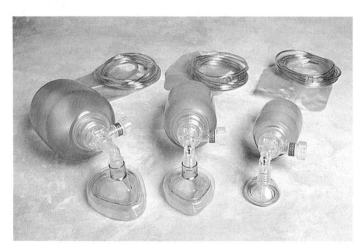

FIGURE 6-17 Different sizes of bag valve mask (BVM).
© American Academy of Orthopaedic Surgeons.

Masks vary in size and complexity from the simple face shield to the bag valve mask (BVM). Each type of mask has distinct advantages and disadvantages. Because you probably will not have the opportunity of choosing the mask you prefer in an emergency, you should learn how to use all types correctly.

Follow these steps when performing mouth-to-mask rescue breathing:

1. Position yourself at the patient's head.

2. Open the patient's airway using either the head tilt–chin lift or the jaw-thrust maneuver **FIGURE 6-18**.

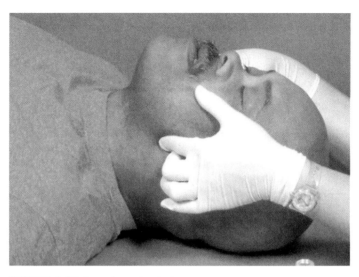

FIGURE 6-18 Open the patient's airway.
© Jones & Bartlett Learning.

3. Place the mask over the patient's mouth and nose.

4. Using both hands, grasp the mask and the patient's jaw. Press down on the mask with your thumbs as you lift up on the jaw with your fingers. This will create a good seal between the mask and the patient's face **FIGURE 6-19**.

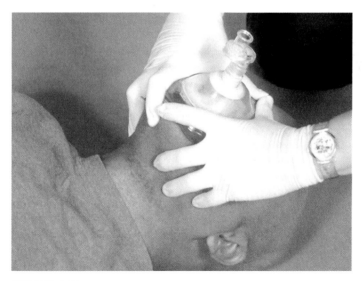

FIGURE 6-19 Seal the mask against the patient's face.
© Jones & Bartlett Learning.

5. Place your mouth over the mouthpiece and perform rescue breathing as described in Chapter 4, *Basic Life Support for Adults and Children* **FIGURE 6-20**.

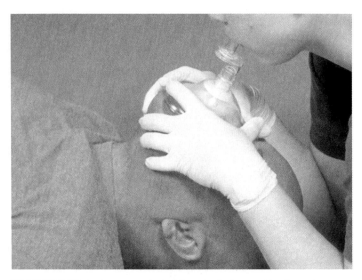

FIGURE 6-20 Seal your mouth over the mouthpiece and begin rescue breathing.
© Jones & Bartlett Learning.

Bag Valve Mask

The BVM is a handheld device with three main components: a bag, a valve, and a mask. The bag is self-inflating; when you squeeze it, it automatically reinflates. The valve is a one-way valve that prevents the patient's exhaled air from entering the bag. The mask is similar to that used for mouth-to-mask rescue breathing. The BVM can be used with an oral and/or a nasal airway. The device delivers a higher concentration of oxygen than a ventilation mask alone—approximately 90% to 100% oxygen when an oxygen source and reservoir are attached to it. Even without supplemental oxygen and an oxygen reservoir, the BVM provides approximately 21% oxygen, which is greater than the 16% oxygen provided by mouth-to-mask rescue breathing.

To use the BVM effectively, you must practice regularly. The best results are achieved when two providers use the device. One provider maintains an open airway and mask-to-face seal, while the second provider squeezes the bag **FIGURE 6-21**. The bag should be squeezed smoothly, not forcefully. Forceful compression, like forceful rescue breathing, will result in more air entering the patient's stomach than the lungs.

Rescue Airway Devices

There are numerous devices that are inserted into the mouth without direct visualization of the vocal cords. These rescue airway devices have been designed to maintain a patent airway and allow for adequate ventilation. The King LT is a single-lumen airway that is blindly inserted into the esophagus. The laryngeal mask airway (LMA), a supraglottic device, features a single lumen with a masklike cuff that protects the airway. The i-gel® supraglottic device is similar to the LMA; however, the mask is made of silicone and expands when placed into the pharynx; it does not have an inflatable mask as does the LMA.

The advantages associated with rescue airway devices include the following:

- They are easy to place (blind insertion).
- No mask seal is needed.
- They offer relative protection against aspiration.

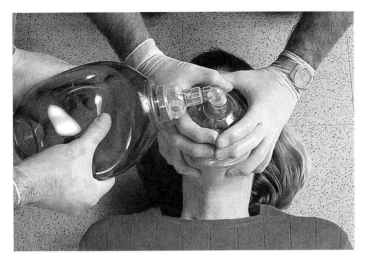

FIGURE 6-21 Two-person bag-valve-mask ventilation.
© Jones & Bartlett Learning. Courtesy of MIEMSS.

The disadvantages associated with rescue airway devices include the following:

- They are ineffective if the cuff malfunctions.
- They require proper assessment of breath sounds.
- They cannot be used on all patients.
- The King LT, LMA, and i-gel® come in various sizes (refer to the manufacturer's guidelines regarding the use of these devices).
- Pediatric sizes are not available for all devices.

The King LT is a single-lumen airway that is blindly inserted into the esophagus **FIGURE 6-22**. It consists of a curved tube with ventilation ports located between two inflatable cuffs. Both cuffs are inflated simultaneously with a syringe that attaches to a single valve. When the airway is properly placed in the esophagus, the distal cuff seals the esophagus; the proximal cuff keeps the tongue off the back of the throat, seals the oropharynx, and prevents air from exiting the patient's mouth during ventilations **FIGURE 6-23**. Openings located between these two cuffs provide ventilation of the lungs once positioning is confirmed.

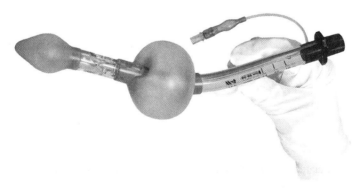

FIGURE 6-22 The King LT is a single-lumen airway that is blindly inserted into the esophagus.
Courtesy of King Systems.

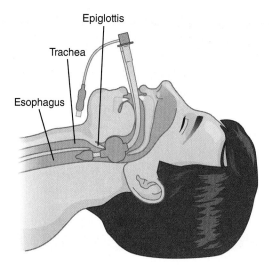

FIGURE 6-23 Placement of the King LT. When properly placed, the distal cuff seals the esophagus and the proximal cuff seals the oropharynx.
© Jones & Bartlett Learning.

The LMA consists of a tube and a masklike cuff at the end. When it is placed correctly, it blocks off the esophagus and allows air to enter the trachea only **FIGURE 6-24**. The LMA is inserted in the mouth and slid down the back of the throat until resistance is met. The masklike cuff is inflated to cover the esophagus, allowing air to go into the trachea.

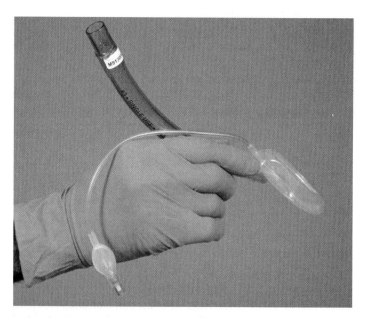

FIGURE 6-24 The laryngeal mask airway (LMA) is an effective rescue airway device.
© Jones & Bartlett Learning. Courtesy of MIEMSS.

The i-gel® consists of a tube and a silicone mask at the end. When correctly placed, it blocks the esophagus and allows air to enter the trachea only **FIGURE 6-25**. The i-gel® is inserted into the mouth and slid down the back of the throat until resistance is met in the same manner as the LMA. Unlike the LMA, however, the silicone mask expands, rather than being inflated with air, to provide a seal in the pharynx **FIGURE 6-26**.

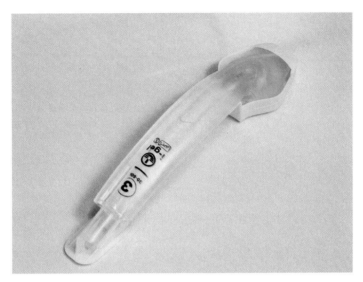

FIGURE 6-25 The i-gel® supraglottic airway device.
© Photo Researchers, Inc./Science Source.

SOFT SKILL

Know Your Equipment

It is critical to maintain a solid working knowledge of every piece of equipment that you may use during a resuscitation. Furthermore, you should check your equipment on a regular basis to ensure that it is fully functional. Do *not* wait until an emergency to try to figure out how a piece of equipment works.

Endotracheal Intubation

Health care providers must be aware of the risks, benefits, and indications for inserting an endotracheal tube (ET) during resuscitative efforts. Unlike the rescue airway devices previously discussed, the ET tube is designed to enter the trachea and directly facilitate ventilation; a distal cuff is then inflated in order to prevent fluids from entering the lungs (aspiration). The ET tube may be a better alternative to other airway devices in certain situations. Insertion of an ET tube—as with any advanced airway device—should *not* interrupt chest compressions. The health care provider who inserts the ET tube should be skilled in advanced airway management.

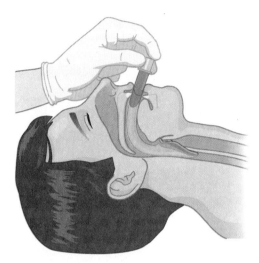

FIGURE 6-26 Correct position of the i-gel® in the airway.
© Jones & Bartlett Learning.

Once an ET tube—or any advanced airway device (eg, King LT, LMA, i-gel®)—is in place during cardiac arrest, you should deliver continuous chest compressions at a rate of 100 to 120 per minute and ventilations at a rate of 10 breaths per minute (1 breath every 6 seconds). Do not attempt to synchronize compressions and ventilations; there should not be a pause in chest compressions to deliver a ventilation.

Confirmation of Advanced Airway Placement

Health care providers should perform a thorough assessment after an advanced airway device has been inserted to verify correct placement. Assessment should include visualization of chest rise, presence of bilateral breath sounds, the absence of sounds over the epigastrium (stomach), and quantitative waveform capnography. These techniques should be used continuously throughout any resuscitation attempt. When transferring or moving the patient, you should confirm that the advanced airway did not dislodge.

Quantitative waveform capnography is the recommended method of confirming initial advanced airway placement, as well as monitoring ongoing advanced airway placement. Capnography measures the amount of carbon dioxide (CO_2) during the exhalation phase; this is referred to as end-tidal CO_2 ($ETCO_2$). It provides real-time objective data via a light-emitting diode (LED) reading and a visible waveform on the cardiac monitor/defibrillator. After inserting the advanced airway, an adapter is placed between the airway device and BVM, with a filter line that connects to the cardiac monitor/defibrillator. The health care provider can then continuously monitor the LED reading and waveform.

Circulatory Assist Devices

Impedance Threshold Devices

An impedance threshold device (ITD) is a valve device placed between the ET tube and a BVM; it may also be placed between the bag and the mask if an ET tube is not in place. The ITD is designed to limit the air entering the lungs during the recoil phase between chest compressions **FIGURE 6-27**. This results in negative intrathoracic pressure that may draw more blood toward the heart, ultimately resulting in improved cardiac filling and circulation during each chest compression. The ITD may be considered when used together with devices that provide active compression–decompression cardiopulmonary resuscitation (CPR). It is *not* currently recommended for use with conventional CPR. If return of spontaneous circulation occurs, then the ITD should be removed. You should understand research trends regarding the effectiveness of the ITD.

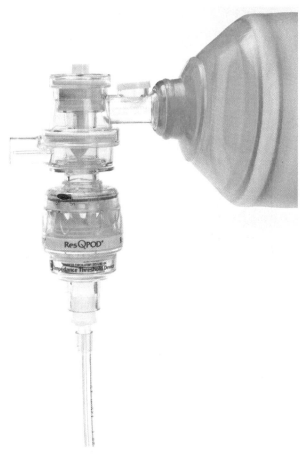

FIGURE 6-27 Impedance threshold device.
Courtesy of Advanced Circulatory Systems, Inc.

Active Compression–Decompression CPR

Active compression–decompression CPR is a technique that involves compressing the chest and then actively pulling it back up to its neutral position or beyond (decompression). This technique may increase the amount of blood that returns to the heart and, thus, the amount of blood ejected from the heart during the compression phase. The active compression–decompression CPR device features a suction cup that is placed in the center of the chest **FIGURE 6-28**. After compressing the chest to the proper depth, the rescuer pulls up on the handle of the device to provide active decompression of the chest, thus ensuring that the chest returns to at least its neutral position, or even beyond neutral.

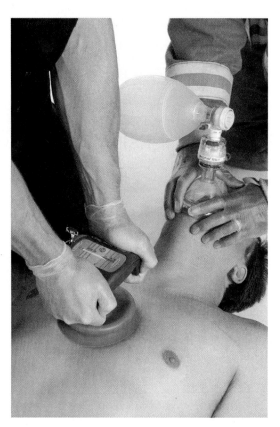

FIGURE 6-28 An active compression–decompression CPR device.
Provided with permission by ZOLL Medical.

Mechanical CPR Devices

Mechanical devices in theory may provide better vital organ blood flow and increased blood pressure in comparison with manual CPR **FIGURE 6-29**. These devices include a load-distributing band (vest) and a mechanical piston device. Although a mechanical CPR device may be a reasonable alternative when personnel and resources are limited, it should be noted that manual CPR remains the standard of care.

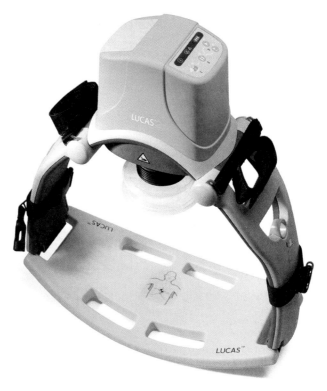

FIGURE 6-29 A mechanical CPR device.
Courtesy of LUCAS CPR (Physio Control Inc.).

Automated External Defibrillation

The most common initial rhythm seen in sudden cardiac arrest (SCA) is ventricular fibrillation (VF)—an abnormal rhythm in which the cardiac electrical conduction system is in a state of chaos, resulting in an uncoordinated "quivering" of the heart muscle and the absence of a pulse. The most important factors for surviving SCA are immediate high-quality CPR and early defibrillation. By applying defibrillator pads to the chest and delivering a shock, you may be able to reestablish a normal cardiac rhythm. In the defibrillation process, a direct electrical current is passed through the heart to momentarily stop all electrical activity. The earlier this occurs, the better the chance that the heart's normal pacemaker cells will take command of the heart's electrical activity and produce a coordinated, regular rhythm and heartbeat.

The time frame from SCA to defibrillation is a crucial factor in determining survival. The earlier defibrillation can be performed, the greater a patient's chance of survival. The likelihood of survival decreases rapidly over time as VF persists. After 8 to 10 minutes of cardiac arrest, damage to the heart and brain are often so extensive that the patient cannot survive **FIGURE 6-30**.

Although not all patients undergoing cardiac arrest will need defibrillation, most adults who experience SCA will be in VF—a condition that is corrected with defibrillation. For this reason, national efforts have been made to advocate placing low-cost, easy-to-use automated external defibrillators (AEDs) where they will be most useful. AEDs are commonly found in places of mass gatherings—stadiums, shopping malls, factories, schools, and aircraft—so they can be used quickly when the need arises. Many law enforcement officers and fire department vehicles also carry AEDs.

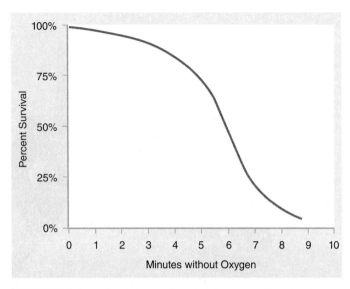

FIGURE 6-30 A patient's chance of survival decreases with each minute that passes without treatment.
© Jones & Bartlett Learning.

FYI

Compression-Only CPR

Health care providers should advocate for communitywide compression-only CPR training and public access defibrillation programs in their respective communities. The perception still exists that bystander CPR involves *both* chest compressions and mouth-to-mouth rescue breathing; this is not true. Bystanders are often hesitant to provide assistance, out of fear of either being sued or contracting a disease. The health care provider should consider it a professional responsibility to educate the public that compression-only CPR and rapid defibrillation with an AED are critical to the patient's survival.

The Heart's Electrical Conduction System

The normal pacemaker for the heart is the sinoatrial (SA) node. Approximately every second, it emits an electrical impulse that travels along pathways through the atria, causing them to contract. This signal is received at the atrioventricular (AV) node, between the atria and the ventricles. The AV node acts as a relay station. Below it, the electrical pathway divides into two main branches—called bundle branches—which serve the two ventricles. When the electrical impulse reaches the Purkinje fibers in the ventricles, it causes the muscular walls of the ventricles to contract. This ventricular contraction forces blood to surge from the heart throughout the body, resulting in a pulse that can be felt at the carotid, brachial, and radial arteries **FIGURE 6-31**.

Abnormal Electrical Activity

Normal and abnormal cardiac rhythms are interpreted using an electrocardiogram (ECG). Although ECG interpretation is an advanced level skill, the provider should have a basic understanding of lethal cardiac rhythms. A normal cardiac rhythm is seen in **FIGURE 6-32**. VF occurs when irregular electrical impulses originate from multiple sites in the ventricles. The heart muscle reacts erratically, trying to respond to too many signals. A chaotic ventricular rhythm results in the fibrillation, or quivering, of the ventricles instead of a regular, strong contraction **FIGURE 6-33**. VF does not produce blood flow from the heart.

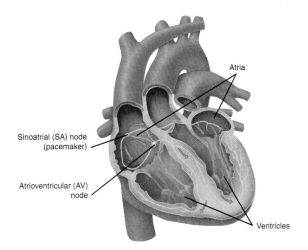

FIGURE 6-31 Cross-sectional view of the heart and its conduction system.
© Jones & Bartlett Learning.

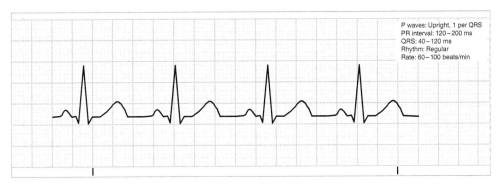

FIGURE 6-32 Normal electrocardiogram (ECG) tracing.
Adapted from Arrhythmia Recognition: The Art of Interpretation, courtesy of Tomas B. Garcia, MD.

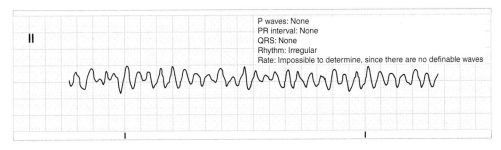

FIGURE 6-33 Ventricular fibrillation.
Adapted from Arrhythmia Recognition: The Art of Interpretation, courtesy of Tomas B.Garcia, MD.

Another abnormal electrical rhythm is ventricular tachycardia (VT). In VT, the heart beats at a rapid rate of between 150 and 200 beats per minute. At this rate, contractions become ineffective and the heart is unable to pump out enough blood **FIGURE 6-34**.

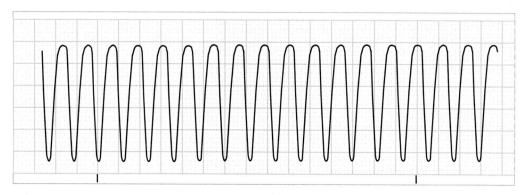

FIGURE 6-34 Ventricular tachycardia.
Adapted from 12-Lead ECG: The Art of Interpretation, courtesy of Tomas B. Garcia, MD.

Automated External Defibrillators

There are many different models of AEDs. The principles are the same for each, but displays, controls, and options may vary. Some AEDs have screens that display the cardiac rhythm and provide verbal prompts; others provide only verbal prompts. Most devices automatically analyze the rhythm, although some older models may require the operator to press a button to begin analysis. There are also different combinations of recording devices for documenting and transferring patient information. The most common AED is the semi-automated defibrillator, which automatically analyzes the patient's heart rhythm but does not automatically deliver a shock; the health care provider initiates the shock after ensuring that no one is touching the patient. Consult the manufacturer's recommendations for the specific model before using it **FIGURE 6-35**.

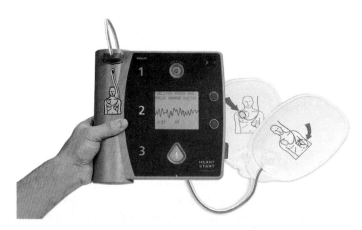

FIGURE 6-35 AEDs have a built-in rhythm analysis system to determine whether the patient needs to be defibrillated.
© Jones & Bartlett Learning. Courtesy of MIEMSS.

The AED is applied only to patients who are in cardiac arrest (ie, unresponsive, not breathing, and pulseless). After confirming that the unresponsive patient is not breathing and does not have a pulse, begin CPR (starting with chest compressions) and apply the AED as soon as it is available. Continue chest compressions while a second rescuer attaches the AED pads. It is essential to avoid delays in chest compressions; frequent and lengthy (longer than 10 seconds) delays in chest compressions decrease the chance of a good patient outcome.

Follow these steps when using an AED:

1. Place the AED near the patient's head and turn it on.

2. Expose the patient's chest and make certain the skin is clean and dry.

3. Remove the backing from the two AED pads and place the pads on the chest according to the manufacturer's directions. Place one pad on the upper right side of the chest just beneath the clavicle. Place the other pad on the left lower ribs, to the left of the nipple. Do *not* interrupt chest compressions when applying the AED pads.

4. Ensure that the electrodes are plugged into the AED.

5. Stop compressions and make sure no one is touching the patient. Allow the AED to analyze the heart rhythm, which may require pushing an "Analyze" button on the AED. If the patient is in VF or VT, the AED will recommend defibrillation.

6. If the AED advises a shock, continue CPR while the defibrillator is charging. (If no shock is advised, resume CPR for 5 cycles [about 2 minutes] and then reanalyze the cardiac rhythm.)

7. Ensure that no one is touching the patient, and deliver the shock.

8. After defibrillation, immediately resume CPR, starting with chest compressions.

9. After five cycles (about 2 minutes) of CPR, stop compressions and allow the AED to reanalyze the rhythm.

10. Repeat steps 5 through 8 until advanced life support (ALS) personnel arrive or the patient starts to move.

If the cables or pads are not secure, the AED will give an error warning (eg, "Check patient"). Likewise, the AED will not analyze the heart rhythm if the patient is moving, which is why it may not be possible to use the device in a moving vehicle, such as the back of an ambulance.

If the AED states "No shock advised," immediately resume CPR, starting with chest compressions, and prepare to transport or transfer the patient. This patient, as well as one who does not respond to defibrillation, needs ALS measures or has suffered too great an injury to the heart to survive.

AED Precautions

When using an AED:

- Do not use alcohol to wipe the patient's chest before applying the pads.
- Do not apply the pads directly over any medication patches, such as nitroglycerin **FIGURE 6-36**. Remove any medication patches with your gloved hand and wipe away any residue before applying the pads.
- Do not apply the pads over any implantable pacemaker or automated implantable cardioverter/defibrillator. Place the pads at least 1 inch (3 cm) away from such devices.
- Do not defibrillate a patient who is lying on a surface likely to conduct electricity (eg, in a puddle of water).
- If the patient's chest is wet, quickly dry it off with a towel before applying the AED pads.
- Do not press the shock button or analyze the rhythm until everyone is clear of the patient.

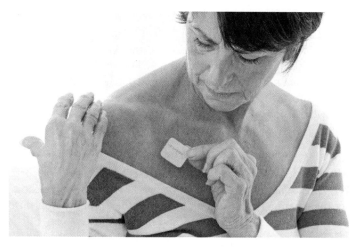

FIGURE 6-36 Any medication patches on the chest, including those for nitroglycerin, must be removed before AED pads are placed.
© BSIP/Science Source.

AED Use in Children

AEDs can safely be used in children younger than 8 years using the pediatric-sized pads and a dose-attenuating system (energy reducer) **FIGURE 6-37**. However, if these devices are unavailable, you should use adult AED pads. An AED should be used as soon as possible for an infant or child with a witnessed arrest. For children with an unwitnessed arrest, the AED should be applied after the first five cycles of CPR have been completed. Cardiac arrest in infants and children is usually the result of respiratory failure; therefore, oxygenation and ventilation are vitally important. After the first five cycles of CPR, the AED should be used to deliver shocks in the same manner as with an adult.

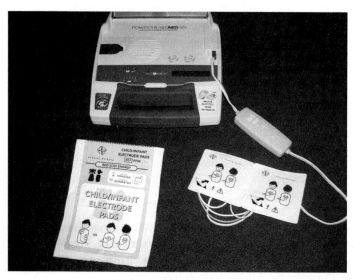

FIGURE 6-37 AED pads for pediatric use.
© Cardiac Science Corporation.

If the child is between 1 month and 1 year of age (an infant), a manual defibrillator is preferred to an AED. However, manual defibrillation is an ALS skill; therefore, you should request ALS support immediately. If ALS personnel with a manual defibrillator are not immediately available, pediatric pads with a dose attenuator (energy reducer) are preferred. If neither is available, use adult AED pads. If you are using adult AED pads on an infant, ensure that the pads are not touching. If necessary, place one pad on the back and the other pad on the chest.

AED Maintenance

AEDs can greatly improve the chance of survival for a person in cardiac arrest if applied quickly and properly. But the device must also function properly when it is applied. To be certain that your AED will function properly when needed, you must inspect it regularly as part of preventive maintenance.

Additionally, expiration dates should be checked on pads and batteries. Proper documentation should be kept on these inspections. If the unit should fail to function during an emergency, your documentation will be very important as the incident is reviewed.

PREP KIT

Ready for Review

- A patient's airway must be clear and open before you can provide rescue breathing. Airway obstructions may be caused by anatomic conditions, such as the tongue blocking the airway; this requires minimal effort to correct. Other times, the airway may be obstructed by foreign material such as food, blood, or vomitus.

- Manual and mechanical suction units are available to help remove debris from the airway. Mechanical suction devices are powered by batteries or pressurized oxygen. Whichever type of suction device you use, it is important to understand the machinery and not to suction too deeply or aggressively.

- Patients can benefit from devices that help you maintain an open airway. If the patient is unconscious and has no gag reflex, you can use an oral or nasal airway device. Select the correct size to avoid triggering a gag reflex or blocking the airway. You may use the nasal airway device on semiconscious patients and/or those who have an active gag reflex; however, do not use the nasal airway in patients with a suspected skull or nasal fracture.

- Various devices, such as simple ventilation masks or bag valve masks (BVMs), are available to support ventilation and reduce the risk of disease transmission. With supplemental oxygen attached, the BVM can deliver between 90% and 100% oxygen to the patient. Advanced airway devices designed to facilitate airway management and ventilation include the endotracheal (ET) tube and supraglottic airways, such as the King LT, laryngeal mask airway (LMA), and i-gel®.

- Early CPR and defibrillation have consistently been shown to save lives for people with SCA. The indications for using an AED are that the patient is unresponsive, not breathing, and pulseless. If you are caring for a patient in cardiac arrest, begin CPR (starting with chest compressions) and apply the AED as soon as it is available.

PREP KIT continued

- Once turned on and attached to the patient's bare chest, the AED will analyze the heart's rhythm and advise whether or not a shock is indicated. If a shock is advised, ensure that no one is touching the patient, deliver the shock, and immediately resume CPR (starting with chest compressions). Perform CPR for 2 minutes and reanalyze the patient's heart rhythm. If no shock is advised, perform CPR for 2 minutes and then reanalyze the patient's rhythm. Continue CPR and rhythm analysis until ALS personnel arrive or the patient starts to move.

Vital Vocabulary

active compression–decompression CPR A technique for delivering chest compressions that involves compressing the chest and then actively pulling it back up to its neutral position or beyond (decompression).

aspiration In the context of the airway, the introduction of vomitus or other foreign material into the lungs.

atrioventricular (AV) node A point between the atria and ventricles that sends electrical impulses to the ventricles.

automated external defibrillator (AED) A device that analyzes a patient's heart rhythm, recognizes the presence of ventricular fibrillation and pulseless ventricular tachycardia, and advises the health care provider to deliver a shock.

bag valve mask (BVM) A ventilation device with a face mask attached to a bag with a reservoir and oxygen connection that delivers between 90% and 100% oxygen to the patient.

defibrillation Use of a special electrical current in an attempt to convert a fibrillating (chaotically beating) heart to a normal, rhythmic beat.

end-tidal CO_2 ($ETCO_2$) The amount of carbon dioxide present in exhaled breath.

impedance threshold device (ITD) A valve device that is placed between the endotracheal tube and a bag valve mask or between the bag

and the mask if an endotracheal tube is not in place. It is designed to limit the air entering the lungs during the recoil phase between chest compressions, with the net effect of drawing more blood back to the heart.

nasopharyngeal (nasal) airway An artificial airway adjunct that is inserted through a nostril of a person who has a gag reflex.

oropharyngeal (oral) airway An artificial airway adjunct that is inserted into the mouth of an unconscious patient without a gag reflex to keep the tongue from obstructing the airway.

Purkinje fibers Conduction pathways through the ventricles.

quantitative waveform capnography A system to measure the amount of carbon dioxide during the exhalation phase of respiration. It provides real-time objective data via a light-emitting diode (LED) reading and a visible waveform on the cardiac monitor/ defibrillator and is used to confirm and monitor correct placement of an advanced airway device.

rescue airway devices Advanced airway devices that are blindly inserted to secure an open airway and allow for ventilation of the lungs. Types include the King LT, laryngeal mask airway (LMA), and i-gel.

septum The partition between the nostrils.

sinoatrial (SA) node A site containing the heart's primary pacemaker.

PREP KIT continued

ventilation masks Masks of various sizes and complexities that are designed to help ventilate patients while offering some protection from potentially infectious body fluids.

ventricular fibrillation (VF) An abnormal rhythm in which the cardiac electrical conduction system is in a state of chaos,

resulting in an uncoordinated "quivering" of the heart muscle and the absence of a pulse; treated with defibrillation.

ventricular tachycardia (VT) A rapid, regular heart rhythm that often does not produce effective cardiac output; may deteriorate to ventricular fibrillation.

Check Your Knowledge

1. In which of the following patients should you insert an oropharyngeal (oral) airway?

   A. Any unconscious patient without a gag reflex

   B. Semiconscious patient with shallow breathing

   C. Unconscious patient with an intact gag reflex

   D. Semiconscious patient with a skull or nasal fracture

2. The safest and MOST effective method for providing rescue breathing to a nonbreathing patient is the:

   A. one-person bag-valve-mask technique.

   B. mouth-to-mouth technique.

   C. mouth-to-mask technique.

   D. two-person bag-valve-mask technique.

3. When ventilating a nonbreathing patient with a bag valve mask, you can deliver the highest concentration of oxygen to the patient by:

   A. squeezing the bag forcefully.

   B. attaching an oxygen reservoir.

   C. keeping the airway slightly flexed.

   D. delivering 20 to 24 breaths per minute.

4. A nasopharyngeal (nasal) airway should NOT be used on a patient who:

   A. may have a skull or nasal fracture.

   B. is semiconscious with a gag reflex.

   C. gags when you insert an oral airway.

   D. is unconscious without a gag reflex.

5. Which of the following statements regarding the use of an AED in children is correct?

   A. It is too dangerous to use adult AED pads in children between the ages of 1 and 8 years.

   B. The AED cannot be used in infants because defibrillation may cause excessive heart damage.

   C. Currently, there is no evidence to support the safe use of AEDs in children.

   D. Pediatric-sized pads and a dose attenuator are preferred in children younger than 8 years.

6. After confirming that an adult patient is in cardiac arrest, you should:

   A. give two rescue breaths and start chest compressions until an AED arrives, has been applied, and is ready to analyze.

   B. begin CPR only after you have applied an AED and analyzed the heart rhythm.

   C. perform CPR, starting with chest compressions, until an AED arrives, has been applied, and is ready to analyze.

   D. perform CPR for 3 minutes before applying an AED.

7. You have applied the AED to a patient in cardiac arrest and have received a "Shock advised" message. After ensuring that no one is touching the patient and delivering the shock, you should:

   A. check for a carotid pulse for no longer than 10 seconds.

   B. resume CPR, starting with chest compressions, for 2 minutes.

   C. wait at least 3 minutes before defibrillating the patient again.

   D. reanalyze the heart rhythm to confirm that a shock is advised.

8. The health care provider should NOT use an AED on a patient who:

   A. is in a puddle of water or on a wet sidewalk.

   B. has a nitroglycerin patch on their chest.

   C. has an implanted pacemaker or defibrillator.

   D. experienced an unwitnessed cardiac arrest.

9. After inserting an advanced airway device in a patient who is in cardiac arrest, you should:

   A. ventilate the patient between 20 and 24 times per minute.

   B. stop after every 30 chest compressions to give a breath.

   C. decrease the chest compression rate to at least 80 per minute.

   D. avoid synchronizing chest compressions and ventilations.

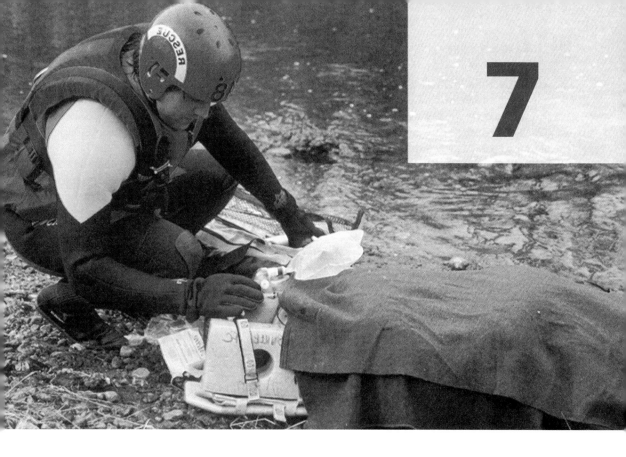

Special Resuscitation Situations

Working With Special Challenges

Some emergency situations present special challenges for the health care provider. Although the initial basic life support procedures still apply, special situations such as trauma, drowning, hypothermia, electrocution, pregnancy, opioid overdose, and anaphylaxis require additional skills.

Trauma

According to the Centers for Disease Control and Prevention, unintentional injuries are the leading cause of death for people 1 to 44 years of age. To have the best chance of survival, a patient with serious trauma from a severe physical injury should be transported to the most appropriate hospital, which should be a trauma center, for specialized treatment. In some cases, it may be necessary to transport a patient to the closest hospital for immediate stabilization if a trauma center is located far away. Even with the best care possible, however, some trauma patients do not survive. This is especially true of trauma patients who experience cardiac arrest at the scene.

Whenever you encounter an unresponsive person, you must consider the possibility that they have sustained a head or neck injury. This consideration is particularly important for trauma patients injured by violent actions such as falls, motor vehicle collisions, or diving-related incidents. If the patient is conscious, you should perform a careful assessment to look for signs and symptoms of a head or neck injury.

A common cause of unresponsiveness is brain injury, but any serious head injury may be accompanied by injury to the patient's spine. Signs and symptoms of spinal cord injury include (Note: Some of these will not be detectable in an unresponsive patient):

- Numbness, tingling, or weakness in the arms or legs
- Loss of bowel or bladder control
- Paralysis of the arms or legs

Care of Trauma Patients

The care you provide to trauma patients begins with the ABCs (airway, breathing, and circulation). Start by carefully positioning the patient, keeping the head in line with the body if you need to roll them. Any unresponsive trauma patient's airway should be opened with the jaw-thrust maneuver; however, if the jaw thrust does not adequately open the patient's airway, carefully perform a head tilt–chin lift maneuver. If you must move the patient quickly due to an unsafe environment, drag the patient, headfirst, by their clothing to minimize the likelihood of additional injury **FIGURE 7-1**. If the patient is not wearing any clothes, grasp them under the armpits. Support the head on your forearms.

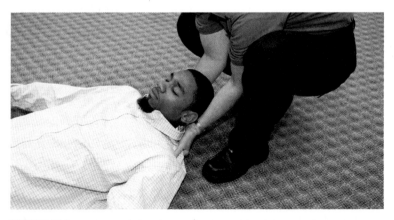

FIGURE 7-1 Emergency clothes drag.
© Jones & Bartlett Learning. Courtesy of MIEMSS.

> **SOFT SKILL**
>
> **Critical Thinking**
>
> It is not uncommon for medical and trauma emergencies to exist in the same patient at the same time. For example, a patient may experience a heart attack, lose consciousness, and run off the road and hit a tree. On the surface, the primary problem may seem to be a traumatic injury. However, what appears obvious may be the least life-threatening problem. Many things can be happening to the patient at the same time, but always address life-threatening problems—airway, breathing, and circulation—before attempting to resolve other issues.

Drowning

Drowning is defined as submersion in water resulting in death within 24 hours. According to the Centers for Disease Control and Prevention, approximately 12 people die from unintentional drowning every day, making it the 6th leading cause of unintentional death in the United States. Near drowning refers to survival for more than 24 hours following submersion. For every person who drowns, it is estimated that four more are hospitalized for near drowning.

Water Rescue

If the person is in the water when you arrive, you can attempt a rescue in one of four ways. Before attempting any water rescue, however, take precautions for your own safety. Never enter deep or moving water without the proper training, equipment, and personnel.

The four ways you can attempt a rescue are easily remembered with the saying—reach, throw, row, go.

1. *Reach* the person with an object such as a pole and hook. Make sure you have secure footing, and have someone grasp your belt or pants to keep you from being pulled in.

2. *Throw* the person something that floats if they are out of reach. A throw bag, life jacket, or flotation cushion will do. Be sure to attach a line to the object so you can pull the person in after they grasp the object **FIGURE 7-2**.

3. *Row*, or use a motorized boat, to reach a person who is out of throwing range. Wear a personal flotation device whenever you enter a boat. Pull the person into the boat when it is safe to do so.

4. *Go* to the person if the water is shallow and there is no danger to you. If the water is deep or swift moving, you must have the necessary equipment, training, and support personnel for a safe rescue.

Care of Drowning Patients

A person who is submerged should be removed from the water as soon as possible to provide the most appropriate care. Although rescue breathing can be done in the water (as long as it does not

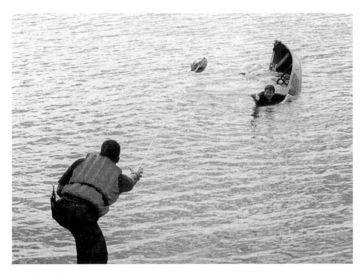

FIGURE 7-2 Throwing assist.
© American Academy of Orthopaedic Surgeons.

compromise rescuer safety), chest compressions and defibrillation require the patient to be removed from the water.

Survival is uncommon in patients who have been submerged for prolonged periods of time; however, successful resuscitation with full recovery has occurred with prolonged submersion—particularly in cold water. Therefore, resuscitation should be attempted unless obvious signs of death are present (eg, decomposition, dismemberment).

After removing the patient from the water, assess them as you would any unresponsive patient. If the patient is not breathing and does not have a pulse, begin CPR (starting with chest compressions) until a defibrillator is available. If the patient is not breathing but has a pulse, provide rescue breathing. If the chest does not visibly rise with your initial ventilation, reposition the head and reattempt to ventilate. If both attempts to ventilate do not produce chest rise, the airway is likely obstructed. Begin airway obstruction removal techniques (eg, chest compressions, looking inside the mouth for obstructions, attempt to ventilate). (See Chapter 4, *Basic Life Support for Adults and Children*, and Chapter 5, *Basic Life Support for Infants*, for more on airway obstruction removal.)

Hypothermia

Hypothermia occurs when the body's core temperature falls below 95°F (35°C). Immersion in cold water, exposure to cold weather, or prolonged exposure to cool, damp conditions can make the body's core temperature drop. It does not need to be very cold for hypothermia to occur. In fact, water that is under 70°F (21°C) can lead to hypothermia. Older adults, young children, and those who are intoxicated are particularly susceptible to this condition. In rare cases, people have survived extended periods of time without a pulse or breathing when their core temperature has fallen below 86°F (30°C). For this reason, it is important to attempt resuscitation even in extreme cases.

The signs and symptoms of hypothermia can be difficult to recognize. Contrary to common belief, the development of hypothermia does not require freezing temperatures. Prolonged exposure to temperatures of 50°F (10°C) can result in hypothermia, particularly if the conditions are humid, rainy, or windy. Suspect severe hypothermia if you note these signs:

- Mental status that changes from disorientation, apathy, or aggressiveness to unresponsiveness.
- Lack of shivering. As the core body temperature drops and the patient becomes less responsive, shivering stops.
- Cool abdomen. The patient's abdomen beneath their clothing is cool or cold to the touch.
- Stiff, rigid muscles, similar to rigor mortis.
- Pallor or cyanosis.

Care of Patients With Hypothermia

If you suspect hypothermia, move the patient to a warmer area, remove wet clothing, and cover the patient with layered blankets to prevent further heat loss **FIGURE 7-3**. Be sure to cover the patient's head; this part of the body is a source of significant heat loss. When positioning the patient, do not raise the legs. Raising the legs causes cold blood from the legs to flow to the body's core. Because severe hypothermia may dramatically slow the heart rate and breathing, the patient may appear to be dead. Therefore, assess breathing and pulse for 30 to 45 seconds before initiating CPR. Abnormal electrical activity (dysrhythmias) may also develop in the heart. Handle the patient gently. Rough handling can cause cardiac arrest in a patient with hypothermia who has a slow pulse.

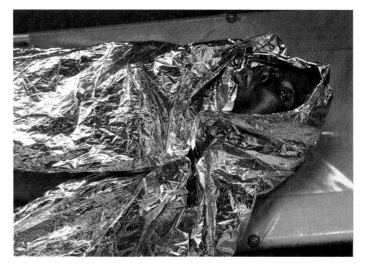

FIGURE 7-3 Aluminized covers or blankets reduce body heat loss.
© ton koene/Alamy Stock Photo.

If the patient with hypothermia is in cardiac arrest, begin CPR until a defibrillator has been applied and ready to analyze the cardiac rhythm—just as you would with any other patient. If the automated external defibrillator (AED) advises you to deliver a shock, deliver one shock and then immediately resume CPR. If the patient does not respond to one shock, continue high-quality CPR, keep the patient warm, and transport to an appropriate medical facility for more aggressive rewarming. Continue to defibrillate, as needed, every 2 minutes during attempts to rewarm the patient.

Patients With Hypothermia

Patients with hypothermia should not be considered dead until they have been appropriately re-warmed, unless signs of obvious death are present.

Electrocution

Safety

Hundreds of people die each year from electrocution, including lightning strikes. Although high voltage is clearly dangerous, deaths have been reported with household current of 110 volts or less. Safety is the most important consideration in dealing with electrocution. When you arrive at a scene involving electrical hazards, take the following safety precautions:

- If you are outside, look for downed power lines before approaching the patient. Count the wires from pole to pole to make sure none are missing. Use a flashlight if it is dark. If the scene is not safe, stay clear and summon other professional resources, including the power company, for assistance.
- If you are inside, unplug or disconnect appliances and lights or turn off the power at the circuit breaker or fuse box.
- If you feel a tingling in your legs and lower body, *stop your approach*. An electrical current is passing up one leg and down the other. Shuffle away with small steps. Be sure to keep your feet together to minimize the possibility of a strong electric shock.
- Do not move wires. Any material, even wood, can conduct a fatal amount of electricity if the voltage is high enough.

During electrocution, electricity passes through the body along the path of least resistance, usually the nerves and/or blood vessels. The current may leave characteristic entrance and exit wounds, but internal damage may not be readily apparent **FIGURE 7-4**. A severe shock may also cause skeletal injuries, such as fractures. Any current may cause the heart to stop beating and go into ventricular fibrillation. If this is the case, proceed with resuscitation when there is no longer any danger of electrocution.

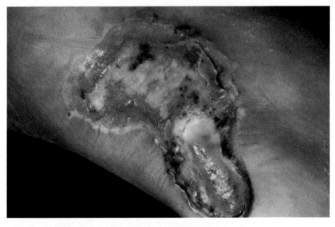

FIGURE 7-4 Exit wound from an electrical burn.
© Charles Stewart MD, EMDM MPH.

A lightning strike is a form of electrocution. People who have been struck by lightning may have burn wounds indicating the path of the current or fractures from the force of the current. Most deaths from lightning are due to cardiac arrest. Those who sustain a lightning strike without experiencing cardiac arrest usually survive.

Care of Electrocution Patients

The possibility of respiratory or cardiac arrest is your primary concern for a person who has been electrocuted. If the patient is in cardiac arrest, the heart rhythm is likely to be ventricular fibrillation, which can be reversed with early CPR and defibrillation. Because massive electrical injuries can cause fractures—including those of the spinal column—open the unresponsive patient's airway with the jaw-thrust maneuver. If the patient is in respiratory arrest, provide rescue breathing. If the patient is in cardiac arrest, begin CPR until a defibrillator is available. Unless associated with major bleeding, care for external burn wounds associated with the electrocution has a low priority for the patient in cardiac arrest.

Maternal Cardiac Arrest

If you encounter a pregnant patient who is in cardiac arrest, then your priorities are to provide high-quality CPR and relieve pressure off the aorta and inferior vena cava. When the patient lies supine, the pregnant uterus can compress the aorta and inferior vena cava (aortocaval compression). Compression of the inferior vena cava causes a significant decrease in blood return to the heart and, subsequently, in the forward flow of blood to the vital organs.

Care of Maternal Cardiac Arrest

If the pregnant patient is not in cardiac arrest, then position her on her left side to relieve pressure on the large blood vessels. However, if she is in cardiac arrest, then this approach is impractical because she must remain in a supine position to maximize the effectiveness of chest compressions. If the top of the patient's uterus (fundus) can be felt at or above the level of the umbilicus, perform manual displacement of the uterus to the left to relieve compression to the aorta and other large blood vessels while CPR is being performed. This step will improve the effectiveness of compressions **FIGURE 7-5**. While one person performs manual displacement of the uterus and a second performs CPR, a third rescuer or bystander should be sent to retrieve an AED.

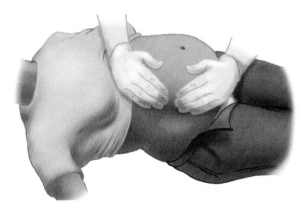

FIGURE 7-5 Manual left displacement of the uterus. The two-handed technique is shown. Alternatively, one hand can be used.
© Jones & Bartlett Learning.

Opioid Overdose

An opioid is a narcotic drug that, when taken in excess, depresses the central nervous system and causes respiratory arrest followed by cardiac arrest. Examples of opioids include heroin, oxycodone, and fentanyl.

Care of Patients Experiencing Opioid Overdose

In situations where opioid overdose is the suspected cause of a patient's cardiac arrest, bystanders may have administered naloxone (Narcan) to the patient prior to the health care provider's arrival. Naloxone blocks opiate receptors in the body and reverses the effect of opioid overdose. Naloxone autoinjector devices and intranasal spray devices, intended for use by laypeople (as well as health care providers), are now available in the United States. If a bystander administered naloxone before your arrival, you should determine how much was given and the route by which it was given. The recommended algorithm for implementing naloxone into the cardiac arrest management sequence is shown in **FIGURE 7-6**.

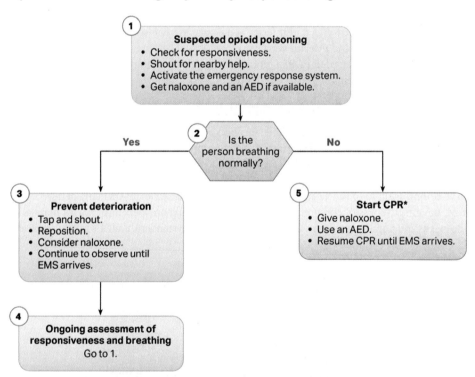

Opioid-Associated Emergency for Lay Responders Algorithm

1 **Suspected opioid poisoning**
- Check for responsiveness.
- Shout for nearby help.
- Activate the emergency response system.
- Get naloxone and an AED if available.

2 Is the person breathing normally?

Yes

3 **Prevent deterioration**
- Tap and shout.
- Reposition.
- Consider naloxone.
- Continue to observe until EMS arrives.

4 **Ongoing assessment of responsiveness and breathing**
Go to 1.

No

5 **Start CPR***
- Give naloxone.
- Use an AED.
- Resume CPR until EMS arrives.

*For adult and adolescent victims, responders should perform compressions and rescue breaths for opioid-associated emergencies if they are trained and perform Hands-Only CPR if not trained to perform rescue breaths. For infants and children, CPR should include compressions with rescue breaths.

© 2020 American Heart Association

FIGURE 7-6 Recommended algorithm for treating cardiac arrest caused by opioid overdose.
Reprinted with permission Circulation.2020;142:S366-S468 ©2020 American Heart Association, Inc

Standard resuscitative measures (ie, high-quality chest compressions, ventilation, defibrillation) take priority over naloxone administration. Do not delay these critical interventions in order to administer naloxone. Many patients who have overdosed on an opioid have a pulse (although slow) but are not breathing. In these patients, artificial ventilation is the most critical treatment, followed by administration of naloxone if it is available.

FYI

Patients Experiencing Opioid Overdose in Cardiac Arrest

Oxygenation and ventilation through rescue breathing are the most important treatments for an unresponsive patient who is apneic (or has abnormal breathing) following an opioid overdose. Restore effective oxygenation and ventilation first, then consider administering naloxone.

There is no proven benefit to administering naloxone to patients in cardiac arrest—even if their cardiac arrest was caused by an opioid overdose. In these cases, focus your efforts on high-quality CPR and defibrillation (if indicated). Administer naloxone if directed by your local protocols.

Anaphylaxis

Anaphylaxis, also called anaphylactic shock, is a severe allergic reaction that is caused by an exaggerated immune system response to a foreign substance. In anaphylaxis, the immune system releases chemicals into the bloodstream following exposure to something that the patient is allergic to (eg, insect venom, medication). These chemicals cause swelling of the upper airway, narrowing of the bronchioles in the lungs, and systemic dilation of the blood vessels. Signs and symptoms of anaphylaxis include:

- Difficulty breathing
- High-pitched sound during inhalation (stridor)
- Low blood pressure (hypotension)
- Widespread hives (urticaria)

Care of Patients With Anaphylaxis

Anaphylaxis does not resolve on its own. Without prompt treatment, the patient will die of respiratory and/or circulatory system failure. The lifesaving treatment for anaphylaxis is epinephrine. Epinephrine dilates the bronchioles in the lungs (improves breathing) and constricts the systemic blood vessels (increases blood pressure).

Patients with known allergies to insect venom, medications, and other agents *should* carry an epinephrine autoinjector with them at all times. The health care provider can assist the patient with their autoinjector if needed. If the patient does not have an autoinjector, the health care provider can draw up epinephrine from a vial or ampule, if properly trained and authorized by local protocol. The recommended dose is 0.2 to 0.5 mg (1:1,000 solution), which is administered via the intramuscular route.

PREP KIT

Ready for Review

- Special resuscitation situations include trauma, drowning, hypothermia, electrocution, maternal cardiac arrest, and opioid overdose. These situations present you with special challenges when providing care. Remember that trauma patients may have experienced spinal injuries; therefore, caution must be used when moving them.

- When water rescue is needed, you should attempt it in this order: reach, throw, row, and go. Never attempt a water rescue unless you have special training and equipment for this type of rescue. Consider the possibility of spinal injury in anyone found unresponsive in the water, especially shallow water. Clear the patient's airway before beginning resuscitation. Unless obvious signs of death are present, attempt resuscitation—even if the person has been submerged for a prolonged period of time. This is especially important if the patient was rescued from cold water.

- Hypothermia may occur with patients who have been submerged in cool or cold water and in other situations besides extremely cold weather. Because severe hypothermia dramatically slows the heart rate and breathing, assess the patient's breathing and pulse for 30 to 45 seconds before initiating CPR. Handle patients with hypothermia gently; they are at greater risk for cardiac arrest.

- When dealing with electrocution, make sure there is no longer any danger of electrical injury to you or the patient. Your first consideration in an electrocution emergency is your own safety. Do not attempt to gain access to the patient until the scene is safe. Assume that patients may have serious internal injuries, even if entrance and exit wounds are small. Because electrocution injuries cause massive muscle spasms and spinal fractures, you should also suspect a possible spinal cord injury.

- When caring for a pregnant patient who is in cardiac arrest, your priorities are to provide high-quality CPR and to relieve pressure off the venae cavae and aorta. If the top of the uterus (fundus) is above the level of the umbilicus, manually displace the uterus to the patient's left side.

- Opioid overdose can cause respiratory arrest, followed by cardiac arrest. If the patient is apneic or is breathing abnormally, rescue breathing is the most important immediate treatment, followed by naloxone (Narcan). Naloxone autoinjector and intranasal spray devices are intended for bystander use but can also be used by health care providers. If the patient is in cardiac arrest, focus your efforts on high-quality CPR and defibrillation (if indicated). Although there is no proven benefit to giving naloxone to patients in cardiac arrest—even if the arrest was caused by an opioid overdose—your local protocols may advocate its administration.

- Anaphylaxis is an imminently life-threatening emergency that requires immediate treatment with epinephrine, either via autoinjector or intramuscular injection.

PREP KIT continued

Vital Vocabulary

anaphylaxis A severe allergic reaction caused by an exaggerated immune system response to a foreign substance, such as insect venom or a medication, to which the patient is allergic.

aorta The main artery that receives blood from the left ventricle of the heart and delivers it to all the other arteries that carry blood to the tissues of the body.

drowning Death from suffocation within 24 hours following submersion in water.

fundus The dome-shaped top of the uterus.

hypothermia An abnormally low body temperature.

naloxone A drug used to counteract the effects of opioids; trade name Narcan.

near drowning Survival for at least 24 hours following submersion in water.

opioid Any synthetic narcotic drug that affects the opiate receptors in the brain.

uterus The muscular organ where the fetus grows, also called the womb; responsible for contractions during labor.

Check Your Knowledge

1. The patient with serious trauma has the best chance of survival if they:

   A. are kept warm with blankets.

   B. are transported to a trauma center.

   C. receive oxygen as soon as possible.

   D. receive early advanced life support.

2. A water rescue should not be attempted until:

   A. you determine how long the patient has been in the water.

   B. the patient has been asked if they can swim to the shore.

   C. you have taken proper precautions to ensure your own safety.

   D. Advanced life support personnel have been summoned and have arrived at the scene.

3. When treating a patient with severe hypothermia and cardiac arrest, you should:

   A. defibrillate every 2 minutes as needed.

   B. perform chest compressions at a slower rate.

   C. avoid any attempts at rewarming the patient.

   D. perform compressions but not rescue breaths.

4. When caring for a patient with hypothermia, your initial action should be to:

   A. open the airway with the jaw-thrust maneuver.

   B. move the patient to a warmer area.

   C. check for a pulse for 30 to 45 seconds.

   D. perform a full head-to-toe assessment.

PREP KIT continued

5. Which of the following statements regarding electrical injuries is correct?

   A. Electricity often takes the path of greatest resistance.

   B. External wounds are a good indicator of internal injury.

   C. Ventricular fibrillation is rare following an electrocution.

   D. Deaths have been reported with a current of 110 volts or less.

Evaluation Forms

Start Time: _____ Date: _____

Stop Time: _____

Candidate's Name: _____

Evaluator's Name: _____

One-Person Adult and Child CPR

No.	Task Steps	Satisfactory	Unsatisfactory
1.	Check responsiveness.		
2.	If unresponsive and you are without a mobile phone, shout for help or have someone activate the code team or EMS system.		
3.	Simultaneously check for breathing and a carotid pulse; take no more than 10 seconds.		
4.	If breathing is absent or abnormal but pulse is present, perform rescue breathing (1 breath every 6 seconds for an adult; 1 breath every 2 to 3 seconds for a child).		
5.	If breathing and pulse are absent, give 30 chest compressions at a rate of 100 to 120 per minute.		
6.	Open the airway and give 2 breaths (1 second each).		
7.	If the patient is a child, activate the code team or the EMS system (if not already done) after 5 cycles (about 2 minutes) of CPR. Then return to the child and continue CPR.		
8.	Continue cycles of CPR until an AED arrives or the patient starts to move.		

Retest Approved By: _____ Retest Evaluator: _____

Evaluator Comments: _____

_____

_____

_____

_____

Start Time: _____ Date: _____

Stop Time: _____

Candidate's Name: _____

Evaluator's Name: _____

Two-Person Adult and Child CPR

No.	Task Steps	Satisfactory	Unsatisfactory
1.	Check responsiveness.		
2.	If unresponsive and you are without a mobile phone, send someone to activate the code team or EMS system.		
3.	Simultaneously check for breathing and a carotid pulse; take no more than 10 seconds.		
4.	If breathing is absent or abnormal but pulse is present, perform rescue breathing (1 breath every 6 seconds for an adult; 1 breath every 2 to 3 seconds for a child).		
5.	If breathing and pulse are absent, provider 1 gives 30 chest compressions (adult) or 15 chest compressions (child) at a rate of 100 to 120 per minute.		
6.	Provider 2 opens the airway and gives 2 breaths (1 second each) during the brief pause in chest compressions.		
7.	After 5 cycles (about 2 minutes) of CPR, providers switch roles.		
8.	Continue cycles of CPR until an AED arrives or the patient starts to move.		

Retest Approved By: _____ Retest Evaluator: _____

Evaluator Comments: _____

_____

_____

_____

_____

Start Time: _____   Date: _____

Stop Time: _____

Candidate's Name: _____

Evaluator's Name: _____

Responsive Adult or Child Airway Obstruction

No.	Task Steps	Satisfactory	Unsatisfactory
1.	Determine if the patient is choking by asking, "Are you choking?"		
2.	If the patient nods yes and cannot talk, give abdominal thrusts until the obstruction is relieved or the patient becomes unconscious.		
If the patient becomes unconscious:			
1.	Place the patient in a supine position on the ground.		
2.	Shout for help or have someone activate the code team or EMS system.		
3.	Perform chest compressions (30 chest compressions if you are alone; 15 chest compressions if 2 providers are present and the patient is a child).		
4.	Open the airway and look inside the mouth.		
5.	If a foreign body is visible and can easily be removed, remove it with your fingers and attempt to ventilate.		
6.	If a foreign body is not visible in the mouth, resume chest compressions.		
7.	If alone, activate the code team or EMS system (if not already done) after 5 cycles (about 2 minutes) of CPR. Then return to the patient and resume CPR.		
8.	Continue the sequence of performing chest compressions, opening the airway, and looking inside the mouth until the obstruction is relieved or ALS personnel arrive.		

Retest Approved By: _____   Retest Evaluator: _____

Evaluator Comments: _____

_____

_____

_____

_____

Start Time: _____ Date: _____

Stop Time: _____

Candidate's Name: _____

Evaluator's Name: _____

Unresponsive Adult or Child Airway Obstruction

No.	Task Steps	Satisfactory	Unsatisfactory
1.	Check responsiveness.		
2.	If unresponsive and you are without a mobile phone, shout for help or have someone activate the code team or EMS system.		
3.	Simultaneously check for breathing and a carotid pulse; take no more than 10 seconds.		
4.	If breathing and pulse are absent, perform chest compressions (30 chest compressions if you are alone; 15 chest compressions if 2 providers are present and the patient is a child).		
5.	Open the airway and attempt to ventilate. If the first breath does not produce visible chest rise, reposition the patient's head and reattempt ventilation.		
6.	If both breaths do not produce visible chest rise, resume chest compressions.		
7.	Open the airway and look inside the mouth. If you can see a foreign object and can easily remove it, remove it with your fingers and attempt to ventilate. If you cannot see a foreign object, resume chest compressions.		
8.	If alone, activate the code team or EMS system (if not already done) after 5 cycles (about 2 minutes) of CPR. Then return to the patient and resume CPR.		
9.	Continue the sequence of performing chest compressions, opening the airway, and looking inside the mouth until the obstruction is relieved or ALS personnel arrive.		

Retest Approved By: _____ Retest Evaluator: _____

Evaluator Comments: _____

_____

_____

_____

_____

Start Time: _____ Date: _____

Stop Time: _____

Candidate's Name: _____

Evaluator's Name: _____

One-Person Infant CPR

No.	Task Steps	Satisfactory	Unsatisfactory
1.	Check responsiveness.		
2.	If unresponsive and you are without a mobile phone, shout for help or have someone activate the code team or EMS system.		
3.	Simultaneously check for breathing and a brachial pulse; take no more than 10 seconds.		
4.	If breathing is absent or abnormal but pulse is present, perform rescue breathing (1 breath every 2 to 3 seconds).		
5.	If breathing and pulse are absent (or pulse is less than 60 beats per minute with poor perfusion), give 30 chest compressions at a rate of 100 to 120 per minute.		
6.	Open the airway and give 2 breaths (1 second each).		
7.	After 5 cycles (about 2 minutes) of CPR, activate the code team or EMS system (if not already done). Then return to the infant and resume CPR.		
8.	Continue cycles of CPR until an AED arrives or the patient starts to move.		

Retest Approved By: _____ Retest Evaluator: _____

Evaluator Comments: _____

_____

_____

_____

_____

Start Time: _____ Date: _____

Stop Time: _____

Candidate's Name: _____

Evaluator's Name: _____

Two-Person Infant CPR

No.	Task Steps	Satisfactory	Unsatisfactory
1.	Check responsiveness.		
2.	If unresponsive and you are without a mobile phone, send someone to activate the code team or EMS system.		
3.	Simultaneously check for breathing and a brachial pulse; take no more than 10 seconds.		
4.	If breathing is absent or abnormal but pulse is present, perform rescue breathing (1 breath every 2 to 3 seconds).		
5.	If breathing and pulse are absent (or pulse is less than 60 beats per minute with poor perfusion), provider 1 gives 15 chest compressions at a rate of 100 to 120 per minute.		
6.	Provider 2 opens the airway and gives 2 breaths (1 second each) during the brief pause in chest compressions.		
7.	After 5 cycles (about 2 minutes) of CPR, providers switch roles.		
8.	Continue cycles of CPR until an AED arrives or the patient starts to move.		

Retest Approved By: _____ Retest Evaluator: _____

Evaluator Comments: _____

_____

_____

_____

_____

Start Time: _____ Date: _____

Stop Time: _____

Candidate's Name: _____

Evaluator's Name: _____

Responsive Infant Airway Obstruction

No.	Task Steps	Satisfactory	Unsatisfactory
1.	Determine if the infant is choking. Check for inability to breathe, cough, or cry.		
2.	Give up to 5 back blows and 5 chest thrusts.		
3.	Repeat back blows and chest thrusts until the obstruction is relieved or the patient becomes unconscious.		
If the patient becomes unconscious:			
1.	Position the infant on a firm, flat surface.		
2.	Shout for help or have someone activate the code team or EMS system.		
3.	Perform chest compressions (30 chest compressions if you are alone; 15 chest compressions if 2 providers are present).		
4.	Open the airway and look inside the mouth.		
5.	If a foreign body is visible and can easily be removed, remove it with your fingers and attempt to ventilate.		
6.	If a foreign body is not visible in the mouth, resume chest compressions.		
7.	If alone, activate the code team or EMS system (if not already done) after 5 cycles (about 2 minutes) of CPR. Then return to the patient and resume CPR.		
8.	Continue the sequence of performing chest compressions, opening the airway, and looking inside the mouth until the obstruction is relieved or ALS personnel arrive.		

Retest Approved By: _____ Retest Evaluator: _____

Evaluator Comments: _____

_____

_____

_____

_____

Start Time: _____ Date: _____

Stop Time: _____

Candidate's Name: _____

Evaluator's Name: _____

Unresponsive Infant Airway Obstruction

No.	Task Steps	Satisfactory	Unsatisfactory
1.	Check responsiveness.		
2.	If unresponsive and you are without a mobile phone, shout for help or have someone activate the code team or EMS system.		
3.	Simultaneously check for breathing and a brachial pulse; take no more than 10 seconds.		
4.	If breathing and pulse are absent, perform chest compressions (30 chest compressions if you are alone; 15 chest compressions if 2 providers are present).		
5.	Open the airway and attempt to ventilate. If the first breath does not produce visible chest rise, reposition the patient's head and reattempt ventilation.		
6.	If both breaths do not produce visible chest rise, resume chest compressions.		
7.	If alone, activate the code team or EMS system (if not already done) after 5 cycles (about 2 minutes) of CPR. Then return to the patient and resume CPR.		
8.	Continue the sequence of performing chest compressions, opening the airway, and looking inside the mouth, until the obstruction is relieved or ALS personnel arrive.		

Retest Approved By: _____ Retest Evaluator: _____

Evaluator Comments: _____

_____

_____

_____

_____

Start Time: _____ Date: _____

Stop Time: _____

Candidate's Name: _____

Evaluator's Name: _____

Automated External Defibrillation

No.	Task Steps	Satisfactory	Unsatisfactory
1.	Check responsiveness.		
2.	If unresponsive and you are without a mobile phone, shout for help or have someone activate the code team or EMS system.		
3.	Simultaneously check for breathing and a carotid (adult or child) or brachial (infant) pulse; take no more than 10 seconds.		
4.	If breathing and pulse are absent, perform chest compressions (30 chest compressions if you are alone; 15 chest compressions if 2 providers are present and the patient is an infant or a child).		
5.	Open the airway and give 2 breaths (1 second each).		
6.	Activate the code team or EMS system (if not already done).		
7.	Continue CPR until the AED is available.		
Defibrillation:			
1.	Turn on the AED.		
2.	Ensure a clean/dry skin surface.		
3.	Apply pads to the patient's bare chest. Do not interrupt CPR to do this.		
4.	Plug the electrode connector into the AED.		
5.	Clear the patient.		
6.	Allow the AED to analyze the cardiac rhythm.		
If a shock is indicated:			
1.	Resume chest compressions and push the "Charge" button on the AED. Continue chest compressions while the AED is charging.		
2.	Clear the patient.		
3.	Deliver one shock.		
4.	Immediately resume CPR, starting with chest compressions.		
5.	Reanalyze after 5 cycles (about 2 minutes) of CPR.		
6.	Continue 2-minute cycles of CPR, rhythm analysis, and 1 shock (if indicated) until ALS personnel arrive or the patient starts to move.		

If no shock is indicated:		
1.	Immediately resume CPR, starting with chest compressions.	
2.	Reanalyze after 5 cycles (about 2 minutes) of CPR.	
3.	Continue 2-minute cycles of CPR, rhythm analysis, and 1 shock (if indicated) until ALS personnel arrive or the patient starts to move.	

Retest Approved By: _____ Retest Evaluator: _____

Evaluator Comments: _____

_____

_____

_____

_____

Appendix B

Answer Key

Chapter 1
1. B
2. D
3. A
4. B
5. B

Chapter 2
1. B
2. A
3. B
4. B
5. D

Chapter 3
1. A
2. B
3. A
4. D
5. C

Chapter 4
1. B
2. A
3. B
4. D
5. A
6. B
7. A
8. C
9. D
10. B

Chapter 5
1. B
2. A
3. D
4. D
5. C
6. A
7. B

Chapter 6
1. A
2. D
3. B
4. A
5. D
6. C
7. B
8. A
9. D

Chapter 7
1. B
2. C
3. A
4. B
5. D

Glossary

abdominal thrusts: A method of dislodging food or other foreign material from the throat of a person who is choking and responsive; also known as the *Heimlich maneuver*.

acquired immunodeficiency syndrome (AIDS): A disease in which the body's immune system loses its ability to fight infections and disease processes. It is caused by infection with the human immunodeficiency virus.

active compression–decompression CPR: A technique for delivering chest compressions that involves compressing the chest and then actively pulling it back up to its neutral position or beyond (decompression).

acute coronary syndrome (ACS): A spectrum of clinical disease that refers to unstable angina and acute myocardial infarction (heart attack). The most common symptom is chest pain, pressure, or discomfort.

acute myocardial infarction: Death of a portion of heart muscle caused by a coronary artery occlusion; also known as a heart attack.

advance directive: Written documentation that a competent patient uses to specify medical treatment should that person become unable to make decisions in the future; also called a living will.

advanced cardiac life support (ACLS): The administration of intravenous fluids and medications to help resuscitate a patient experiencing cardiac arrest and prevent a recurrence of cardiac arrest.

airway obstruction: An airway blockage that prevents air from reaching a person's lungs.

alveoli: Air sacs in the lungs where gas exchange takes place.

anaphylaxis: A severe allergic reaction caused by an exaggerated immune system response to a foreign substance, such as insect venom or a medication, to which the patient is allergic.

angina: Chest pain felt when the heart does not receive enough oxygen.

aorta: The main artery that receives blood from the left ventricle of the heart and delivers it to all the other arteries that carry blood to the tissues of the body.

apneic: Absence of spontaneous breathing.

arteries: Blood vessels that carry blood away from the heart.

arterioles: The smallest branches of an artery.

aspiration: In the context of the airway, the introduction of vomitus or other foreign material into the lungs.

atherosclerosis: A disease characterized by a thickening and destruction of the arterial walls, caused by fatty deposits within them; the arteries lose their ability to dilate and carry oxygen-enriched blood.

atria: The two upper heart chambers that receive blood from the body and lungs.

atrioventricular (AV) node: A point between the atria and ventricles that sends electrical impulses to the ventricles.

automated external defibrillator (AED): A device that analyzes a patient's heart rhythm and recognizes the presence of ventricular fibrillation and pulseless ventricular tachycardia; advises the health care provider to deliver a shock.

bag valve mask (BVM): A ventilation device with a face mask attached to a bag with a reservoir and oxygen connection; delivers between 90% and 100% oxygen to the patient.

basic life support (BLS): Noninvasive emergency lifesaving care that is used to treat medical conditions, including airway obstruction, respiratory arrest, and cardiac arrest.

brachial pulse: The pulse found on the inside of the upper arm.

bronchi: The two main air passages that branch out from the trachea.

capillaries: Small blood vessels that connect arterioles and venules and through whose walls various substances pass into and out of the narrow spaces between tissues and then on to the cells.

cardiopulmonary resuscitation (CPR): A method of temporarily circulating oxygenated blood throughout the body of a patient experiencing cardiac arrest. It combines rescue breathing and chest compressions.

cardiovascular disease (CVD): A spectrum of disease processes affecting the heart and circulatory system; the leading cause of death in the United States.

cardiovascular system: System composed of the heart and a complex arrangement of connected tubes (including the arteries, arterioles, capillaries, venules, and veins) that moves blood, oxygen, nutrients, carbon dioxide, and cellular waste throughout the body.

carotid artery: The major artery that supplies blood to the head and brain.

carotid pulse: The pulse felt on the side of the neck, over the carotid artery.

cerebellum: The part of the brain that coordinates body movements.

cerebrum: The largest part of the brain, containing about 75% of the brain's total volume.

chain of survival: A sequence of events that, if performed in a timely manner, can improve survival from cardiac arrest; includes surveillance and prevention, activation of the emergency response system, immediate high-quality CPR, rapid defibrillation, basic and advanced EMS care, advanced life support and postarrest care at the hospital, and recovery of the post cardiac arrest patient.

chest compression fraction: The total percentage of time during a resuscitation attempt in which active chest compressions are being performed.

chest thrusts: A maneuver used to expel objects from the throat of a person who is responsive and has an airway obstruction, particularly infants and patients who are obese or pregnant.

child abuse: Any improper or excessive action that injures or otherwise harms a child or infant; includes neglect and physical, sexual, and emotional abuse.

consent: Permission to treat given by the patient to the health care provider.

coronary arteries: The blood vessels that carry blood and nutrients to the heart muscle.

coronary artery disease (CAD): The presence of atherosclerosis in the coronary arteries, which may cause symptoms such as angina or, ultimately, acute myocardial infarction (heart attack).

coronavirus disease 2019 (COVID-19): The respiratory disease caused by the SARS-CoV-2 virus.

croup: An infectious disease of the upper respiratory system that may cause airway obstruction and is characterized by a barking cough.

cyanosis: A blueness of the skin due to insufficient oxygen in the blood.

defibrillation: Use of a special electrical current in an attempt to convert a fibrillating (chaotically beating) heart to a normal, rhythmic beat.

defibrillator: A device used to deliver a direct current shock to the heart to restore organized cardiac electrical activity.

dependent lividity: Blood settling to the lowest point of the body, causing discoloration of the skin.

diaphragm: A dome-shaped, sheetlike muscle that separates the chest cavity from the abdomen.

drowning: Death from suffocation within 24 hours following submersion in water.

duty to act: The job-defined, legal obligation to provide care.

dysrhythmias: Heart rhythm disturbances caused by abnormal electrical signals sent out by the heart.

electrocardiogram (ECG): A measurement of the electrical impulses generated by the cardiac pacemaker cells.

end-tidal co$_2$ (Etco$_2$): The amount of carbon dioxide present in exhaled breath.

epiglottis: The flaplike cartilaginous structure overhanging the entrance to the trachea that prevents food from entering the trachea during swallowing.

epiglottitis: Inflammation of the epiglottis.

exhalation: The act of breathing out; expiration.

femoral artery: The principal artery of the thigh. It can be palpated in the groin area.

femoral pulse: The pulse felt on the inside of the upper thigh.

fibrinolytic: A medication that can dissolve a clot in a cerebral or coronary artery.

fundus: The dome-shaped top of the uterus.

glottis: The opening to the trachea.

Good Samaritan laws: Laws that protect a person from legal liability when providing emergency care, in good faith, to a suddenly ill or injured person.

head tilt–chin lift maneuver: A procedure for opening the airway in which two movements—tilting back of the forehead and lifting of the chin—are combined.

heart: The hollow muscular organ that receives blood from the veins, sends it through the lungs to be oxygenated, then pumps it to the body via the arteries.

Heimlich maneuver: A method of dislodging food or other foreign material from the throat of a person who is choking and responsive; also known as *abdominal thrusts*.

hepatitis: A viral infection of the liver.

human immunodeficiency virus (HIV): A virus that attacks white blood cells and destroys the body's ability to fight infection. Acquired immunodeficiency syndrome results from HIV infection.

hyperventilation: Rapid or deep breathing that lowers the blood carbon dioxide level below normal.

hypothermia: An abnormally low body temperature.

hypoxia: A dangerous condition in which the body tissues and cells do not have enough oxygen.

impedance threshold device (ITD): A valve device that is placed between the endotracheal tube and a bag valve mask or between the bag and the mask if an endotracheal tube is not in place. It is designed to limit the air entering the lungs during the recoil phase between chest compressions, with the net effect of drawing more blood back to the heart.

implied consent: The assumption that a patient would give consent for treatment if that person were able to do so.

informed consent: Consent to treatment given by the patient who understands the risks and benefits of accepting treatment.

inhalation: The drawing of air into the lungs; inspiration.

intercostal muscles: Muscles between the ribs.

ischemia: A lack of oxygen that deprives tissues of necessary nutrients, resulting from partial or complete blockage of blood flow; potentially reversible because permanent injury has not yet occurred.

jaw-thrust maneuver: A procedure for opening the airway in which the jaw is lifted and pulled forward by placing the index and middle fingers behind the mandible. This keeps the tongue from falling back into the airway; used to open the airway in patients with a suspected spinal injury.

laryngectomy: Surgical removal (partial or complete) of the larynx, usually due to disease of the larynx (ie, cancer).

larynx: The organ of voice production; also called the voice box.

manual defibrillators: Devices that display the patient's cardiac rhythm on a screen and enable the provider to manually select the energy setting before delivering a shock.

medulla oblongata: The part of the brain that is located in the brainstem and that connects the brain to the spinal cord. It controls involuntary functions, such as breathing, heart rate, and digestion.

mild airway obstruction: A condition in which the airway is partially blocked. The patient is able to exchange air in the lungs and cough forcefully but has some degree of respiratory distress.

myocardium: Heart muscle.

naloxone: A drug used to counteract the effects of opioids; trade name Narcan.

nasopharyngeal (nasal) airway: An artificial airway adjunct that is inserted through a nostril of a person who has a gag reflex.

near drowning: Survival for at least 24 hours following submersion in water.

neonate: Person who is age birth to 1 month.

nervous system: The brain, spinal cord, and nerve branches from the central, peripheral, and autonomic nervous systems.

opioid: Any synthetic narcotic drug that affects the opiate receptors in the brain.

oropharyngeal (oral) airway: An artificial airway adjunct that is inserted into the mouth of an unconscious patient without a gag reflex to keep the tongue from obstructing the airway.

pacemaker cells: A mass of specialized muscle fibers in the heart that regulates the electrical function of the heart.

personal protective equipment (PPE): Equipment that protects its wearer, according to standard precautions, from potentially contagious bloodborne or airborne diseases.

pharynx: The portion of the airway between the nasal cavity and the larynx; the throat.

plaque: A substance created by materials in the blood being deposited on the arterial walls.

primary assessment: A step within the patient assessment process that identifies and initiates treatment of immediate and potential life threats.

public access defibrillation (PAD): An initiative that provides training to the public about the importance of early defibrillation and makes automated external defibrillators available in the community for rapid deployment by bystanders.

pulse: The pressure wave that is felt with the expansion and contraction of an artery, consistent with the heartbeat.

Purkinje fibers: Conduction pathways through the ventricles.

quantitative waveform capnography: A system to measure the amount of carbon dioxide during the exhalation phase of respiration. It provides real-time objective data via a light-emitting diode (LED) reading and a visible waveform on the cardiac monitor/ defibrillator and is used to confirm correct placement of an advanced airway device.

radial pulse: The pulse felt on the thumb side of the inner wrist, alongside the radius (radial bone).

recovery position: A position used to maintain a clear airway in an unresponsive patient who is breathing adequately and does not have suspected spinal, hip, or pelvic injuries.

rescue airway devices: Advanced airway devices that are blindly inserted to secure an open airway and allow for ventilation of the lungs. Types include the i-gel, King LT, and laryngeal mask airway (LMA).

rescue breathing: A procedure in which a provider breathes for a patient who is not breathing spontaneously on their own.

respiratory arrest: The cessation of breathing.

respiratory distress: A condition in which respiration becomes compromised from disease, injury, choking, or drowning; results in a limited supply of air to the lungs.

respiratory system: The system of organs that controls the inhalation of oxygen and the exhalation of carbon dioxide.

rigor mortis: Stiffening of the body; a definitive sign of death.

septum: In the heart, the wall separating the left and right sides of the heart. In the nose, the partition between the nostrils.

severe acute respiratory syndrome coronavirus 2 (SARS-CoV-2): The virus that causes an infection called coronavirus disease 2019 (COVID-19), which primarily affects the lungs and can lead to respiratory failure and death.

severe airway obstruction: A condition in which the airway is completely blocked and no air exchange is possible.

sinoatrial (SA) node: The heart's primary pacemaker.

spinal cord: The cord of nerve tissue extending through the center of the spinal column.

standard of care: The quality of care provided to people based on training standards, laws, and national organizations.

standard precautions: An infection control concept and practice that assumes all body fluids are potentially infectious; infectious exposures are dealt with by creating a barrier between the rescuer and the person receiving care.

stoma: An opening in the front of the neck through which a person breathes if the larynx has been surgically removed (laryngectomy).

stridor: A high-pitched sound heard during inhalation; indicates obstruction of the upper airway.

stroke: A rupturing or clogging of the blood vessels that deliver oxygen-rich blood to the brain, depriving the brain of the blood and oxygen it requires.

sudden cardiac arrest (SCA): A condition in which the heart suddenly and unexpectedly stops beating. When this happens, blood stops flowing to the brain and other vital organs; death usually occurs if SCA is not treated within minutes.

sudden unexplained infant death (SUID): Death of an infant (younger than 1 year) that remains unexplained after a complete autopsy and assessment of the scene.

thyroid cartilage: The cartilaginous protuberance in the center of the neck; also referred to as the Adam's apple.

tissue necrosis: Death of tissues due to oxygen deprivation.

trachea: The cartilaginous tube extending from the larynx to its division into the primary bronchi; the windpipe.

tracheal tugging: Collapsing of the trachea, causing it to draw back into the neck.

tuberculosis (TB): A disease affecting the respiratory system that is caused by bacteria that settle in the lungs.

unresponsive: Without awareness; unconscious.

uterus: The muscular organ where the fetus grows, also called the womb; responsible for contractions during labor.

veins: The blood vessels that carry blood from the tissues to the heart.

vena cavae: Two large veins through which blood flows into the right atrium.

ventilation masks: Masks of various sizes and complexities that are designed to help ventilate patients while offering some protection from potentially infectious body fluids.

ventricular fibrillation (VF): An abnormal rhythm in which the cardiac electrical conduction system is in a state of chaos, resulting in an uncoordinated "quivering" of the heart muscle and the absence of a pulse; treated with defibrillation.

ventricular tachycardia (VT): A rapid, regular heart rhythm that often does not produce effective cardiac output; may deteriorate to ventricular fibrillation.

ventricles: The two lower chambers of the heart.

venules: Very small, thin-walled blood vessels.

vertebrae: The 33 bones that make up the spinal column.

Index

Note: Page numbers followed by *f*, *t* denote figures and tables respectively.